U0290626

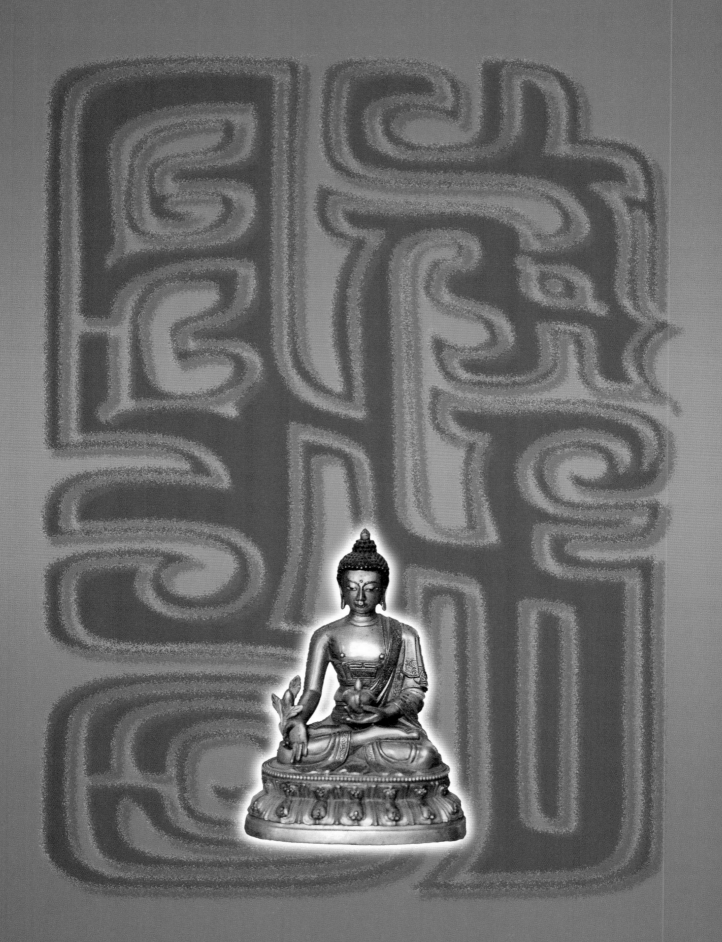

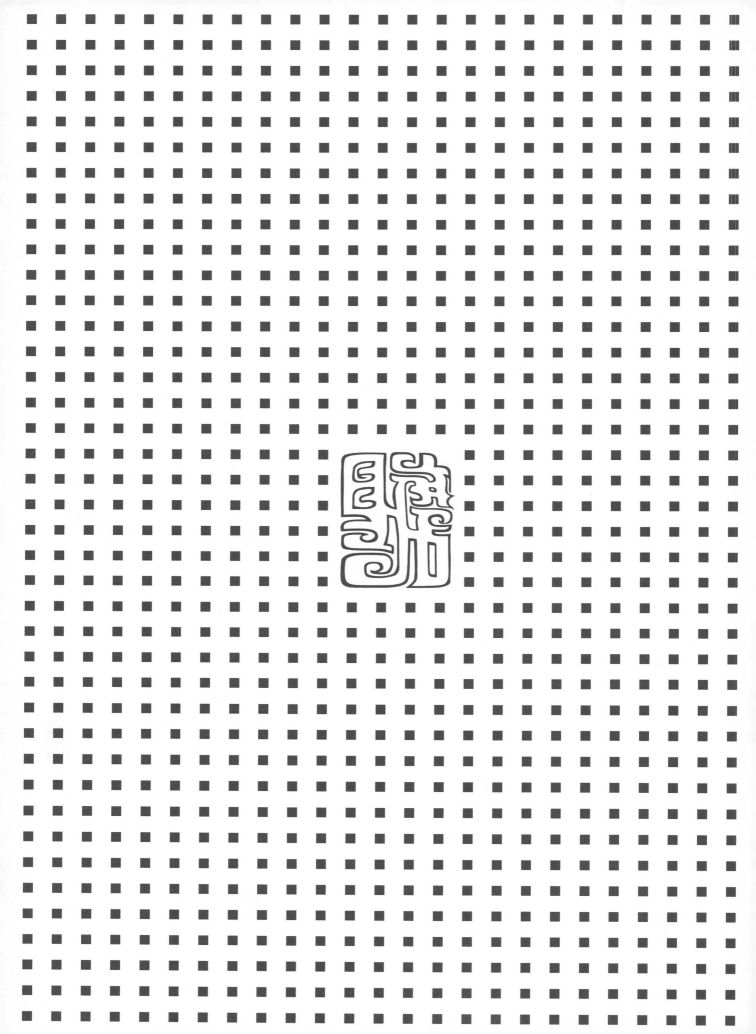

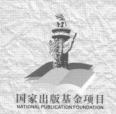

国家出版基金项目
NATIONAL PUBLICATION FOUNDATION

中华医药卫生

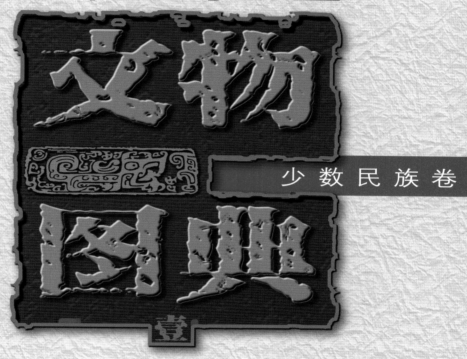

少数民族卷

主　编　李经纬　梁　峻　刘学春
总主译　白永权
主　译　赵永生

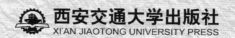

西安交通大学出版社
XI'AN JIAOTONG UNIVERSITY PRESS

图书在版编目（CIP）数据

中华医药卫生文物图典 . 1. 少数民族卷 . / 李经纬，

梁峻，刘学春主编 . — 西安：西安交通大学出版社，2016.12

ISBN 978-7-5605-7018-1

Ⅰ . ①中… Ⅱ . ①李… ②梁… ③刘… Ⅲ . ①中国医药学—

少数民族—文物—中国—图录 Ⅳ . ① R-092 ② K870.2

中国版本图书馆 CIP 数据核字（2015）第 022433 号

书　　名	中华医药卫生文物图典（一）少数民族卷	
主　　编	李经纬　梁　峻　刘学春	
责任编辑	秦金霞	

出版发行　　西安交通大学出版社

　　　　　　（西安市兴庆南路 10 号　邮政编码 710049）

网　　址　http://www.xjtupress.com

电　　话　（029）82668805　82668502（医学分社）

　　　　　　（029）82668315（总编办）

传　　真　（029）82668280

印　　刷　中煤地西安地图制印有限公司

开　　本　889mm×1194mm　1/16　　印张　21.75　　字数　319 千字

版次印次　2017 年 12 月第 1 版　2017 年 12 月第 1 次印刷

书　　号　ISBN 978-7-5605-7018-1

定　　价　680.00 元

读者购书、书店添货、如发现印装质量问题，请通过以下方式联系、调换。

订购热线：（029）82665248　（029）82665249

投稿热线：（029）82668805　（029）82668502

读者信箱：medpress@126.com

版权所有　侵权必究

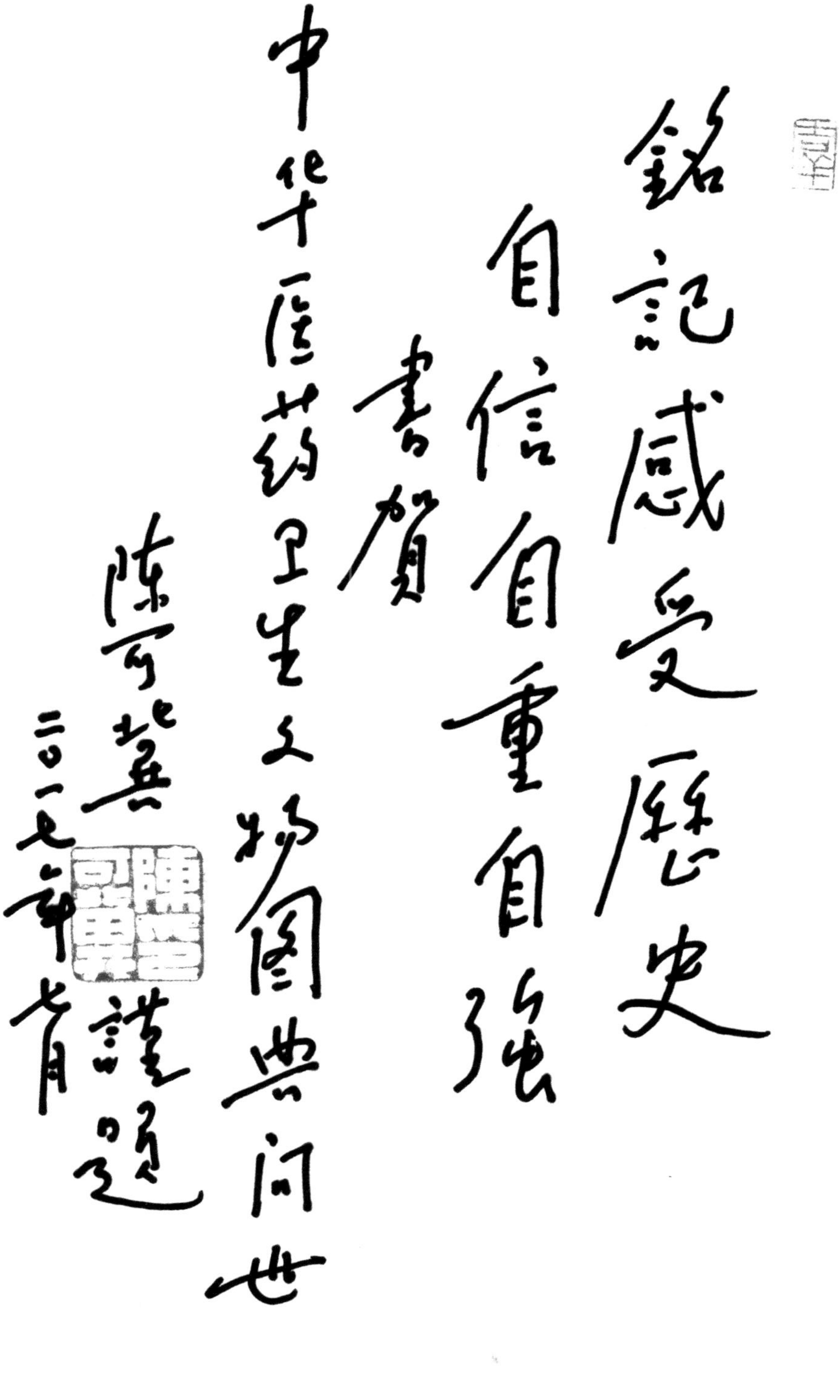

铭记感受历史

自信自重自强

书贺

中华医药卫生文物图典问世

陈可冀 谨题

二〇一七年首月

陈可冀　中国科学院院士、国医大师

精修醫藥衛生文物
圖典功著當代
深究岐黃學術思想
淵源惠澤千秋

中華醫藥衛生文物圖典出版誌慶

丁酉孟秋 孫光榮 敬題於北京

孫光榮　國医大师

中華醫藥衛生文物圖典出版

彰顯中醫藥
文化精神

體現中醫藥
歷史價值

歲次丁酉夏　王琦

王琦　国医大师

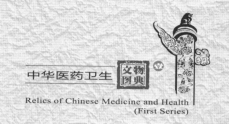

中华医药卫生
文物图典
Relics of Chinese Medicine and Health
(First Series)

中华医药卫生文物图典（一）
丛书编撰委员会

主　编　李经纬　梁　峻　刘学春

副主编　廖　果　吴鸿洲　康兴军　和中浚　刘小斌　杨金生

　　　　郑怀林　徐江雁　白建疆　黄　煌

编　委　李洪晓　梁永宣　王强虎　董树平　马　健　王　霞

　　　　张雅宗　朱德明　包哈申　张建青　郑　蓉　庄乾竹

　　　　李宏红　刘哲峰　王宏才　陈润东

总主译　白永权

主　译　陈向京　聂文信　范晓晖　温　睿　赵永生　杜彦龙

　　　　吉　乐　李小棉　郭　梦　陈　曦

副主译（按姓氏音序排列）

　　　　董艳云　姜雨孜　李建西　刘　慧　马　健　任宝磊

　　　　任　萌　任　莹　王　颀　习通源　谢皖吉　徐素云

　　　　许崇钰　许　梅　詹菊红　赵　菲　邹郝晶

译　者（按姓氏音序排列）

迟征宇　邓　甜　付一豪　高　琛　高　媛　郭　宁

韩　蕾　何宗昌　胡勇强　黄　鋆　蒋新蕾　康晓薇

李静波　刘雅恬　刘妍萌　鲁显生　马　月　牛笑语

唐云鹏　唐臻娜　田　多　铁红玲　佟健一　王　晨

王　丹　王　栋　王　丽　王　媛　王慧敏　王梦杰

王仙先　吴耀均　席　慧　肖国强　许子洋　闫红贤

杨姣姣　姚　晔　张　阳　张　鋆　张继飞　张梦原

张晓谦　赵　欣　赵亚力　郑　青　郑艳华　朱江嵩

朱瑛培

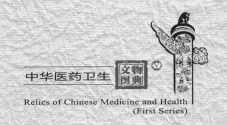

中华医药卫生 文物图典

Relics of Chinese Medicine and Health
(First Series)

本册编撰委员会

主　编　李经纬　梁　峻　刘学春

副主编　廖　果　吴鸿洲　康兴军　和中浚　刘小斌　杨金生

　　　　　郑怀林　徐江雁　白建疆　黄　煌

编　委　李洪晓　梁永宣　王强虎　董树平　马　健　王　霞

　　　　　张雅宗　朱德明　包哈申　张建青　郑　蓉　庄乾竹

　　　　　李宏红　刘哲峰　王宏才　陈润东

总主译　白永权

主　译　赵永生

副主译　许崇钰

译　者　徐素云　铁红玲　邓　甜

丛书策划委员会

丛书总策划　王强虎　王宏才　李　晶　秦金霞

统 筹 人 员　王强虎

丛 书 外 审　王宏才

编辑委员会　王强虎　李　晶　赵文娟　张沛烨　秦金霞　王　磊

　　　　　　　　郭泉泉　郅梦杰　田　滢　张静静

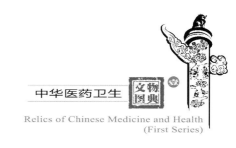

中华医药卫生 文物图典

Relics of Chinese Medicine and Health
(First Series)

序　言

　　探索天、地、人运动变化规律以及"气化物生"过程的相互关系，是人类永恒的课题。宇宙不可逆，地球不可逆，人生不可逆业已成为共识。天地造化形成自然，人类活动构成文化。文物既是文化的载体，又是物化的历史，还是文明的见证。

　　追求健康长寿是人类共同的夙愿。中华民族之所以繁衍昌盛，健康文化起了巨大的推动作用。由于古人谋求生存发展、应对环境变化产生的智慧，大多反映在以医药卫生为核心的健康文化之中，所以，习总书记说："中医药学是中国古代科学的瑰宝，也是打开中华文明宝库的钥匙"。

　　秉持文化大发展、大繁荣理念，中国中医科学院李经纬、梁峻等为负责人的科研团队在完成科技部"国家重点医药卫生文物收集调研和保护"课题获 2005 年度中华中医药学会科技二等奖基础上，又资鉴"夏商周断代工程""中华文明探源工程"等相关考古成果，用有重要价值的新出土文物置换原拍摄质量较差的文物，适当补充民族医药文物，共精选收载 5000 余件。经西安交通大学出版社申报，《中华医药卫生文物图典（一）》（以下简称《图典》）于 2013 年获得了国家出版基金的资助，并经专业翻译团队翻译，使《图典》得以面世。

　　文物承载的信息多元丰富，发掘解读其中蕴藏的智慧并非易事。医药卫生文物更具有特殊性，除文物的一般属性外，还承载着传统医学发展史迹与促进健康的信息。运用历史唯物主义观察发掘文物信息，善于从生活文物中领悟卫生信息，才能准确解读其功能，也才能诠释其在民生健康中的历史作用，收到以古鉴今之效果。"历史是现实的根源"，任何一个民族都不能割断历史，史料都包含在文化中。"文化是民族的血脉，是人民的精神家园"，文化繁荣才能实现中华民族的伟大复兴。值本《图典》付梓之际，用"梳理文化之脉，必获健康之果"作为序言并和作者、读者共勉！

中央文史研究馆馆员
中国工程院院士　　王永炎
丁酉年仲夏

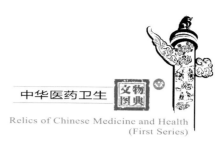

中华医药卫生
文物图典

Relics of Chinese Medicine and Health
(First Series)

前　言

　　文化是相对自然的概念，是考古界常用词汇。文物是文化的重要组成部分，既是文明的物证，又是物化的历史。狭义医药卫生文物是疾病防治模式语境下的解读，而广义医药卫生文物则是躯体、心态、环境适应三维健康模式下的诠释。中华民族是 56 个民族组成的多元一体大家庭，中华医药卫生文物当然包括各民族的健康文化遗存。

　　天地造化如造山、板块漂移、气候变迁、生物起源进化等形成自然。气化物生莫贵于人，即整个生物进化的最高成果是人类自身。广义而言，人类生存思维留下的痕迹即物质财富和精神财富总和构成文化，其一般的物化形式是视觉感知的文物、文献、胜迹等。其中质变标志明晰的文化如文字、文物、城市、礼仪等可称作文明。从唯物史观视角观察，狭义文化即精神财富，尤其体现人类精、气、神状态的事项，其本质也具有特殊物质属性，如量子也具有波粒二相性，这种粒子也是物质，无非运动方式特殊而已。现代所谓可重复验证的"科学"，事实上也是从文化中分离出来的事项，因此也是一种特殊文化形式。追求健康长寿是人类共同的夙愿。中华民族之所以繁衍昌盛，是因为健康文化异彩纷呈。中华优秀传统医药文化之所以博大精深，是因为其原创思维博大、格物致知精深，所以，习总书记说："中医药学是中国古代科学的瑰宝，也是打开中华文明宝库的钥匙"。

文化既反映时代、地域、民族分布、生产资料来源、技术水平等信息，又反映人类认知水平和生存智慧。发掘解读文物、文献中蕴藏的健康知识和灵动智慧，首先是从事健康工作者的责任和义务。《易经》设有"观"卦，人类作为观察者，不仅要积极收藏展陈文物，而且要善于捕捉文物倾诉的信息，汲取养分，启迪思维，收到古为今用之效果。墨子三表法，首先一表即"本之于古者圣王之事"，也是强调古代史实的重要性。"历史是现实的根源"，现实是未来的基础。任何一个国家、地区、民族都不能割断历史、忽略基础，这个基础就是文化。"文化是民族的血脉，是人民的精神家园"。文化繁荣才能驱动各项事业发展，才能实现中华民族的伟大复兴。

人类从类人猿分化出来。"禄丰古猿禄丰种"是云南禄丰发现的类人猿化石，距今七八百万年。距今 200 万年前人类进入旧石器时代，直立行走，打制石器产生工具意识，管理火种，是所谓"燧人氏"时代。中国留存有更新世早、中期的元谋、蓝田、北京人等遗址。距今 10 万—5 万年前，人类进入旧石器时代中期，即早期智人阶段，脑容量增加，和欧洲、非洲人种相比，原始蒙古人种颧骨前突等，是所谓"伏羲氏"时代。中国发现的马坝、长阳、丁村人等较典型。距今 5 万—1 万年前，人类进入旧石器时代晚期，即晚期智人阶段，细石器、骨角器等遍布全国，山顶洞、柳江、资阳人等较典型。

中石器时代距今约 1 万年，是旧石器时代向新石器时代的短暂过渡期，弓箭发明，狗被驯化。河南灵井、陕西沙苑遗址等作为代表。距今 1 万—公元前 2600 年前后，人类进入新石器时代，磨光石器、烧制陶器，出现农业村落并饲养家畜，是所谓"神农氏"时代。公元前 7000 年以来，在甲、骨、陶、石等载体上出现契刻符号、七音阶骨笛乐器等，反映出人文气息趋浓。公元前 6000—公元前 3500 年的老官台、裴李岗、河姆渡、马家浜、仰韶等文化遗址，彰显出先民围绕生存健康问题所做的各种努力。

公元前 4800 年以来，以关中、晋南、豫西为中心形成的仰韶文化，是中原史前文化的重要标志。以半坡、庙底沟类型为典型，自公元前 3500 年走向繁荣，属于锄耕粟黍稻兼营渔猎饲养猪鸡经济方式，彩陶尤其发达。公元前 4400—公元前 3300 年，长江中游的大溪文化，薄胎彩陶和白陶发达。公元前 4300—公元前 2500 年山东丰岛的大汶口文化，红陶为主。公元前 3500 年前后，辽东的红山文化原始宗教发展。公元前 3300 年以来，长江下游由河姆渡、马家浜文化衍续的良渚文化和陇西的马家窑文化、江淮间的薛家岗文化时趋发达。

公元前 2600—公元前 2000 年，黄河中下游龙山文化群形成，冶铸铜器，制作玉器，土坯、石灰、夯筑技术开始应用。公元前 2697 年，轩辕战败炎帝（有说其后裔）、蚩尤而为黄帝纪元元年。黄帝西巡访贤，"至岐见岐伯，引载而归，访于治道"。其引归地"溱洧襟带于前，梅泰环拱于后"，即今河南新密市古城寨。岐黄答问，构建《黄帝内经》健康知识体系，中华文明从关注民生健康起步。颛顼改革宗教，神职人员出现；帝喾修身节用，帝尧和合百国，舜同律度量衡，大禹疏导治水，中华民族不断繁衍昌盛。

公元前 2070 年，禹之子启以豫西晋南为中心建立夏王朝，二里头青铜文化为其特征，半地穴、窑洞、地面建筑并存。饮食卫生器具、酒器增多。朱砂安神作用在宫殿应用。公元前 1600 年，商灭夏。偃师商城设有铸铜作坊。公元前 1300 年，盘庚迁殷，使用甲骨文。武丁时期青铜浑铸、分铸并存。公元前 1056 年，相传周"文王被殷纣拘于羑里，演《周易》，成六十四卦"。公元前 1046 年，武王克商建周，定都镐京。青铜器始铸长篇铭文，周原发掘出微型甲骨文字。公元前 770 年，平王东迁。虢国铸铜柄铁剑。公元前 753 年，秦国设置史官。公元前 707 年出现蝗灾、公元前 613 年出现"哈雷彗星"，均被孔子载入《春秋》。公元前 221 年，秦始皇统一中国，多元一体民族大家庭形成，中华医药卫生文物异彩纷呈。

中国是治史大国，历来重视发展文化博物事业，1955 年成立卫生部中医研究院时就设置医史研究室，1982 年中国医史文献研究所成立时复建中国医史博物馆研究收藏展陈文物。2000—2003 年，经王永炎院士、姚乃礼院长等呼吁，科技部批准立项，由李经纬、梁峻为负责人的团队完成"国家重点医药卫生文物收集调研和保护"项目任务，受到科技部项目验收组专家的高度评价，获中华中医药学会科技进步二等奖。2013 年，在国家出版基金资助下，课题组对部分文物重新拍摄或必要置换、充实民族医药文物后，由西安交通大学出版社编辑、组聘国内一流翻译团队英译说明文字付梓，受到国家中医药博物馆筹备工作领导小组和办公室的高度重视。

"物以类聚"，《图典》主要依据文物质地、种类分为 9 卷，计有陶瓷，金属，纸质，竹木，玉石、织品及标本，壁画石刻及遗址，少数民族文物，其他，备考等卷。同卷下主要根据历史年代或小类分册设章。每卷下的历史时段不求统一。遵循上述规则将《图典》划分为21册，总计收载文物5000余件。对每件文物的描述，除质地、规格、馆藏等基本要素外，重点描述其在民生健康中的作用。对少数暂不明确的事项在括号中注明待考。对引自各博物馆的材料除在文物后列出馆藏外，还在书后再次统一列出馆名或参考书目，以充分尊重其馆藏权，也同时维护本典作者的引用权。

21世纪，围绕人类健康的生命科学将飞速发展，但科学离不开文化，文化离不开文物。发掘文物承载的信息为现实服务，谨引用横渠先生四言之两语："为天地立心，为生民立命"，既作为编撰本《图典》之宗旨，也是我们践行国家"一带一路"倡议的具体努力。希冀通过本《图典》的出版发行，教育国人，提振中华民族精神；走向世界，为人类健康事业贡献力量。

李经纬　梁峻　刘学春

2017年6月于北京

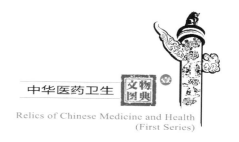

中华医药卫生文物图典

Relics of Chinese Medicine and Health
(First Series)

目 录

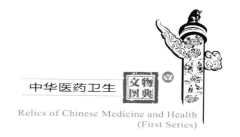

中华医药卫生 文物图典

Relics of Chinese Medicine and Health
(First Series)

Contents

Chapter Five   Textiles

Chapter Six   Paper

Chapter Seven   Miscellanies

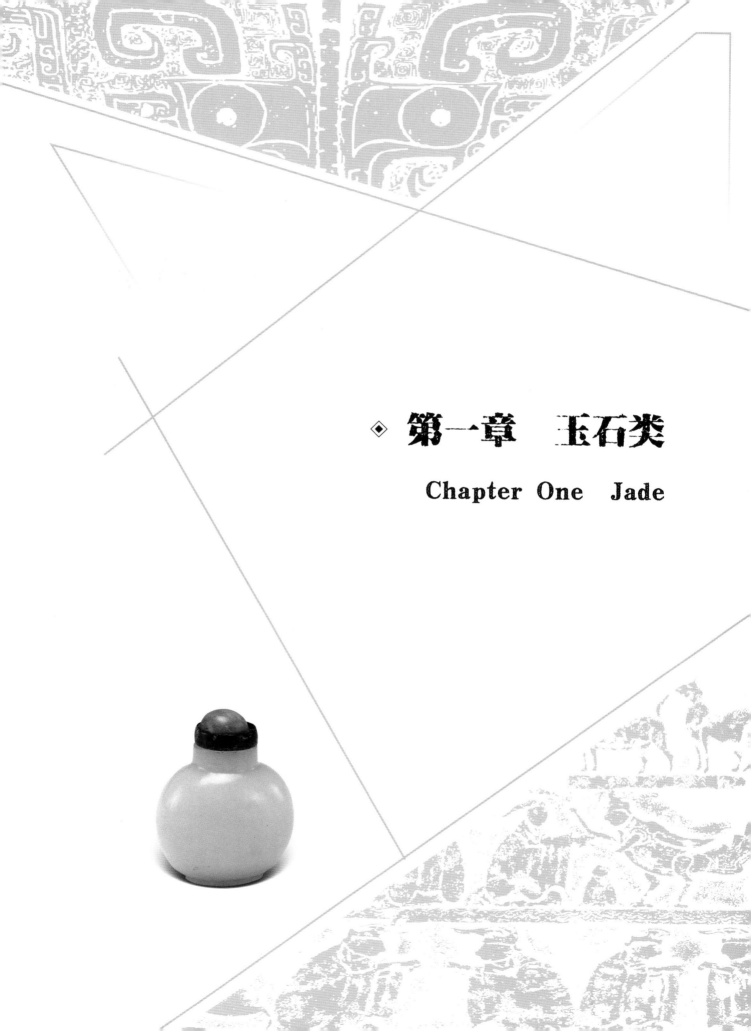

◈ 第一章　玉石类

Chapter One　Jade

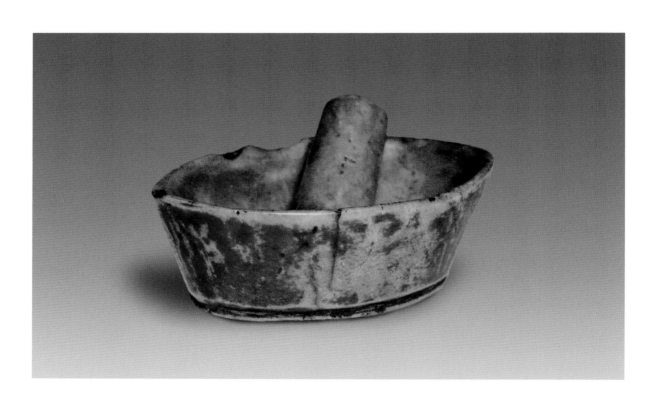

船形玉药臼杵

清

玉质

臼长 18.5 厘米，宽 11 厘米，高 7.5 厘米

杵长 10 厘米

Boat-shaped Jade Mortar and Pestle

Qing Dynasty

Jade

Mortar: Length 18.5 cm/ Width 11 cm/ Height 7.5 cm

Pestle: Length 10 cm

外形像小船，臼内呈枣核圆弧形。此玉药臼杵是新疆莎车维吾尔医院维医依明·阿吉木家传研药用具。新疆莎车征集。

北京中医药大学中医药博物馆藏

The mortar is boat-shaped with an internal arc like a date seed. The mortar and pestle, for porphyrizing drug ingredients, were handed down from the older generations of the family of Yiming Aji, a Uygur doctor in the Uygur Hospital of Shache County, Xinjiang Uygur Autonomous Region. They were collected in Shache County. Preserved in The Museum of Chinese Medicine, Beijing University of Chinese Medicine

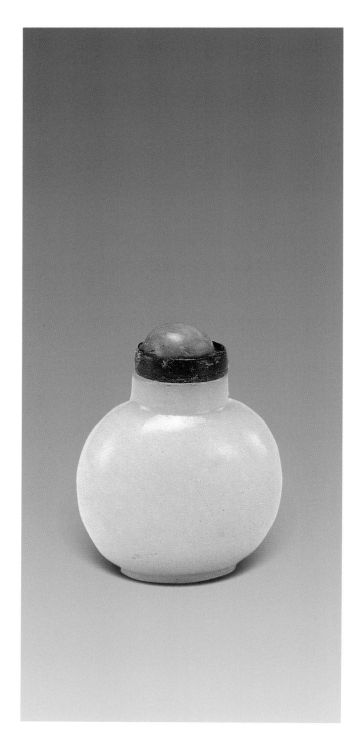

青白玉鼻烟壶

清

玉质

高 6 厘米

用于装药。

内蒙古博物院藏

Light Greenish White Jade Snuff Bottle

Qing Dynasty

Jade

Height 6 cm

It was used to store medicine.

Preserved in Inner Mongolia Museum

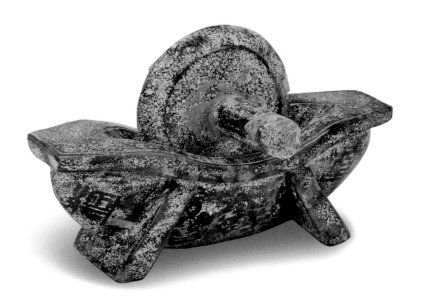

玉石药碾

现代

玉石质

长 25 厘米

用于碾药。

内蒙古国际蒙医蒙药博物馆藏

Jade Medicine Mill

Modern Times

Jade

Length 25 cm

It was used to crush medicine into powder.

Preserved in Inner Mongolia International Mongolian Medicine Museum

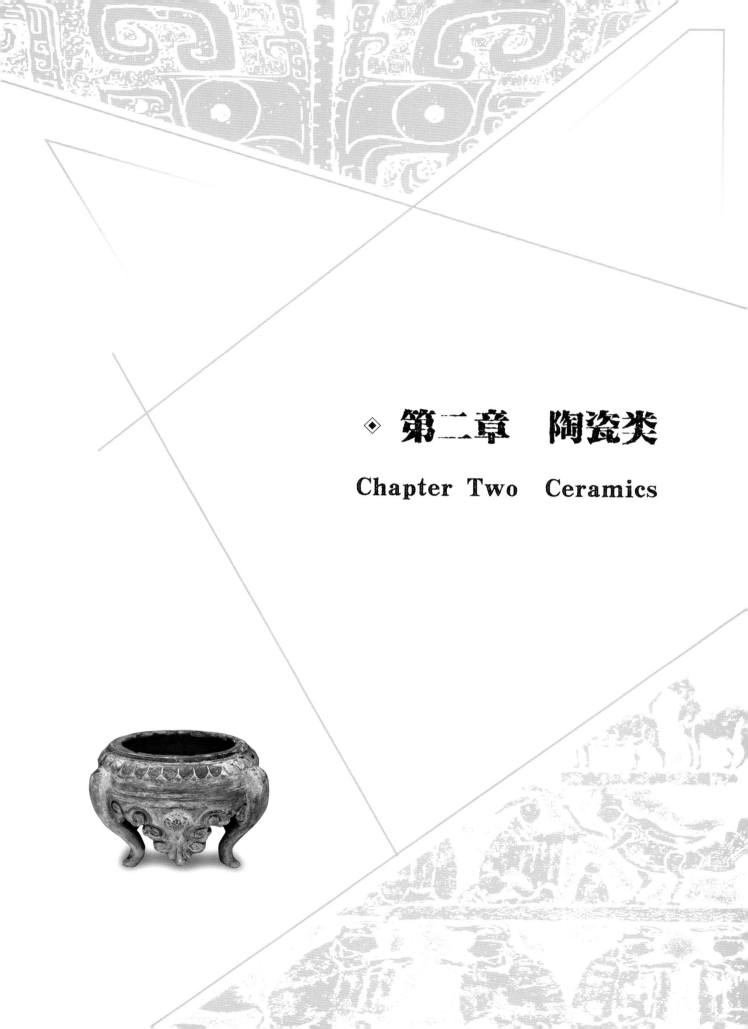

◇ 第二章　陶瓷类

Chapter Two　Ceramics

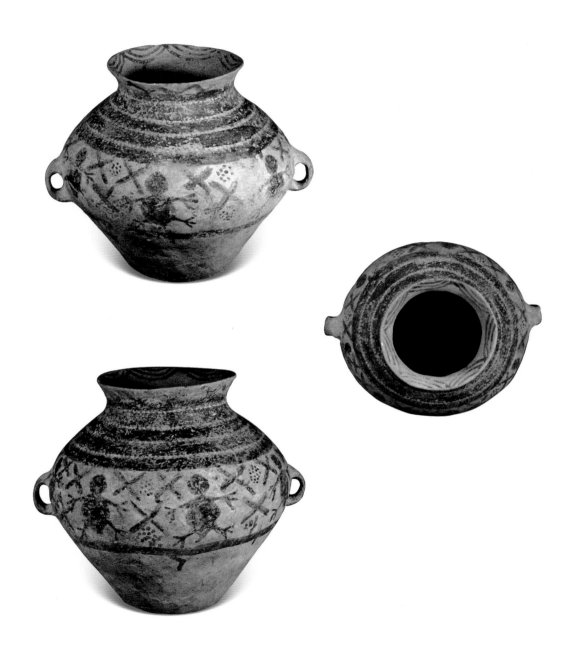

舞蹈孕妇纹陶罐

新石器时代

泥质彩陶

口径 15 厘米，腹径 25 厘米，高 26.5 厘米

胎质厚重，打磨不细，敞口，短颈，溜肩，鼓腹，腹对称环耳，小平底。施黑红双彩，口沿内为连续垂弧纹，颈肩部饰黑宽带锯齿纹与红宽带纹相间，腹部以黑彩饰 7 位舞动的三指孕妇纹。其尾偏向一侧。舞者之间饰蝴蝶纹和圆形点状纹。属马家窑文化边家林类型晚期。

张建青藏

Ceramic Jar with Patterns of Pregnant Women Dancers

The Neolithic Age

Painted Argillaceous Ceramic

Mouth Diameter 15 cm/ Belly Diameter 25 cm/ Height 26.5 cm

The jar uses thick Ceramic and is not well-polished. It has an open mouth, a short neck, declining shoulders, a small flat bottom and a drum-shaped belly on which there are two symmetrical ring ears. It is painted in black and red. On the edge are continuous vertical arc patterns, and on shoulders and the neck are decorated black and red lines of uniform width, and on the belly part are painted 7 dancing pregnant women who have only three fingers. Its bottom leans to one side. There are butterfly lines and round dotted lines between dancers. The pot belongs to the late Bianjialin type of Majia Kiln Culture.

Collected by Zhang Jianqing

神人纹黑红彩罐

新石器时代

泥质黄陶

口径 18 厘米，腹径 37 厘米，高 31 厘米

此罐破裂无缺损，敞口，短颈，圆腹饱满，腹对称环耳，小平底。施黑红双彩，口沿内饰黑垂弧纹和红带纹，颈肩部饰宽带锯齿纹与红带纹。上腹绘四位神人，大头，无五官，内填网纹，上肢曲折向上，三指上托黑色网纹球状物。属马家窑文化半山类型中期。

青海彩陶文化学会提供

Black and Red Colourful Jar with Patterns of Immortals

The Neolithic Age

Yellow Argillaceous Ceramic

Mouth Diameter 18 cm/ Belly Diameter 37 cm/ Height 31 cm

The jar is cracked but has no defect. It has an open mouth, a short neck, a small flat bottom and a drum-shaped belly on which there are two symmetrical ring ears. It is painted in black and red. On the edge is painted in red and black continuous vertical arc patterns, and the shoulders and the neck are decorated with wide black and red zigzag lines. On its upper belly, there are four immortals who have big heads, blank faces filled with net patterns, bending arms upholding black reticulated balls. The pot belongs to the middle Banshan type of Majia Kiln Culture.

Provided by Qinghai Painted Ceramic Culture Society

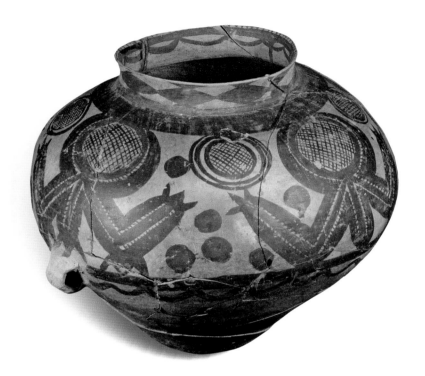

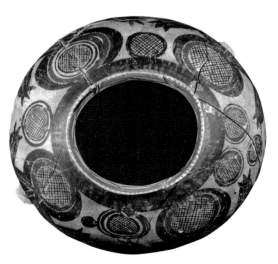

神人纹旋纹鸟形壶

新石器时代

泥质橙黄陶

口径 10.2 厘米，腹径 31.5 厘米，高 26 厘米

此罐破裂修复，短粗颈偏移一侧，先敛后敞形成粗脖子，与颈口对应腹中部有一鋬为尾，腹双环耳为鸟翅。口沿内饰锯齿黑纹和红带纹，颈上部绘网纹，中部画红带纹，根部红带纹之上有大锯齿黑纹，鸟胸前腹为两个大头神人纹手拉着手，头部填绘菱格纹，齐腰部以下为黑带纹和水波纹。属马家窑文化半山类型中期。

青海彩陶文化学会提供

Bird-shaped Pot with Patterns of Immortals

The Neolithic Age

Orange Argillaceous Ceramic

Mouth Diameter 10.2 cm/ Belly Diameter 31.5 cm/ Height 26 cm

This rupture pot has been repaired. It has a stubby neck which is formed by restraining and then extending. Its top mouth has a corresponding protrusion in the belly which is regarded as the tail. Besides, it has two ears in the shape of bird wings. On the edge, there are black zigzag patterns and red band patterns. There are net patterns on the upper neck, red band patterns on the middle neck and big black zigzag patterns above red band patterns on the bottom part of the neck. Two immortals with big heads stand hand in hand on the front belly. Their heads are painted with plaid patterns, and below their waists are black belt lines and water ripple patterns. The pot belongs to the middle Banshan type of Majia Kiln Culture.

Provided by Qinghai Painted Ceramic Culture Society

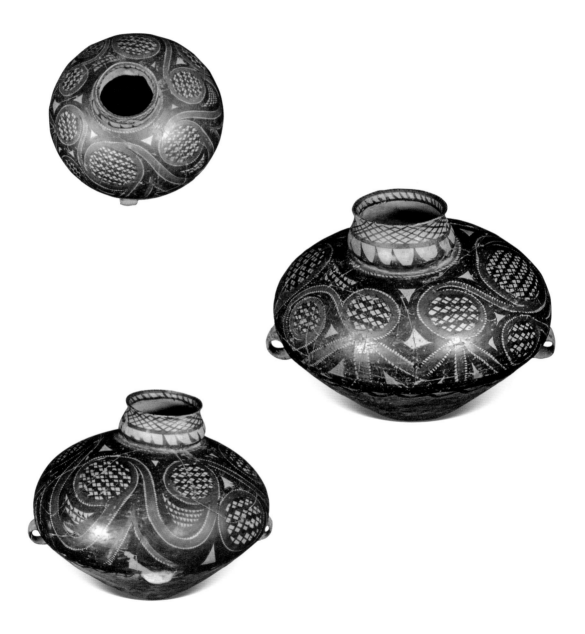

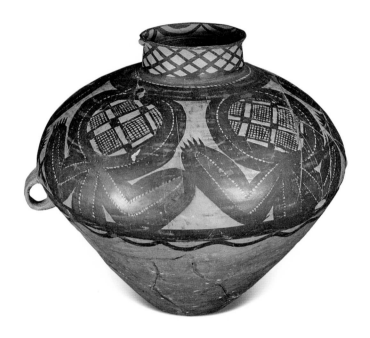

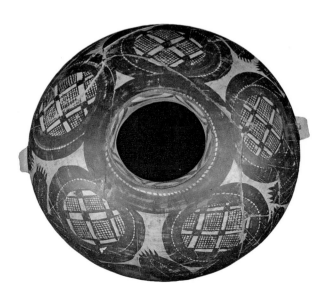

神人纹壶

新石器时代

泥质橙黄陶

口径 13 厘米，腹径 40 厘米，高 40.5 厘米

小敞口，直颈，口沿外对称小盲耳，腹圆呈球形，腹双环耳。施黑红双彩，口沿内饰双垂弧纹，颈上部绘黑红带纹和锯齿纹，腹部绘大头黑红彩神人纹 5 位，以壶口为中心手臂上举，4 至 5 指，下身隐藏于黑色宽带纹和水波纹中。属马家窑文化马厂类型。

青海彩陶文化学会提供

Pot with Patterns of Immortals

The Neolithic Age

Orange Argillaceous Ceramic

Mouth Diameter 13 cm/ Belly Diameter 40 cm/ Height 40.5 cm

The pot has a small open mouth, a straight neck, small blind symmetrical ears along the edge and a round belly with two ears. It is painted in black and red with continuous vertical arc patterns on the edge, wide black and red band and zigzag patterns on the neck. On the belly, there are patterns of five immortals with big heads, upholding arms circling the pot mouth in 4-5 fingers with the lower part of the body hidden under black band patterns and water wave patterns. The pot belongs to the Machang type of Majia Kiln Culture.

Provided by Qinghai Painted Ceramic Culture Society

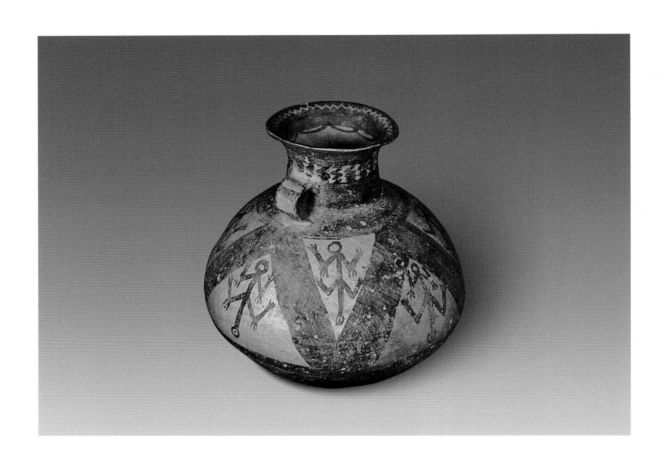

折线神人纹单耳壶

新石器时代

泥质土黄陶

口径 12 厘米，腹径 26.5 厘米，高 27 厘米

Single-eared Pot with Patterns of Curve-lined Immortals

The Neolithic Age

Yellow Argillaceous Ceramic

Mouth Diameter 12 cm/ Belly Diameter 26.5 cm/ Height 27 cm

敞口，中长直颈，颈中一侧至肩有一单环耳，相对下腹部有一錾突，溜肩，垂腹，小平底。施黑红双彩，口沿内饰垂弧纹、红带纹和锯齿纹，颈部绘红带纹和折线纹，腹部画红宽带折线纹，黑彩勾边，俯视为等边四角星，每个折线内绘神人纹1位，共8位，躯干末端饰夸张的女性生殖器官。属马家窑文化马厂类型。

青海彩陶文化学会提供

The pot has an open mouth, a straight long neck, a ring ear on one side of the neck and a protrusion on the lower belly. It has declining shoulders, a vertical belly and a small flat bottom. It is painted in black and red with continuous vertical arc patterns and patterns of red band and zigzag lines on the edge. On the neck there are red band and fold line patterns. And on the belly there are wide red band and fold line patterns outlined in black. When it is overlooked, these patterns form four equilateral angles. Inside each fold line, there are patterns of an immortal whose body end is decorated with exaggerated female genital organs. There are altogether eight immortals. The pot belongs to the Machang type of Majia Kiln Culture.

Provided by Qinghai Painted Ceramic Culture Society

女阴纹壶

新石器时代

泥质土黄陶

口径 13.5 厘米，腹径 35 厘米，高 38.5 厘米

敞口，短颈，腹部两侧各有一环耳，溜肩，垂腹，小平底。施黑彩，口沿内饰梯形纹，其内显示陶色方块纹，口沿外间断折线纹，颈根部绘宽带纹，肩部画大凹凸纹，凹纹内饰小网纹，凸纹内画间隔方块纹，腹部绘 12 个女阴，其中 1 个明显小于其他。属马家窑文化马厂类型。

青海彩陶文化学会提供

Pot with Patterns of Cysthuses

The Neolithic Age

Yellow Argillaceous Ceramic

Mouth Diameter 13.5 cm/ Belly Diameter 35 cm/ Height 38.5 cm

The pot has an open mouth, a short neck, a ring ear on each side of the vertical belly, declining shoulders and a small flat bottom. It is painted in black. There are trapezoidal patterns on its edge, square patterns in Ceramic color inside, fold line patterns outside the edge, wide band patterns on the neck and concavo-convex patterns on the shoulders. There are small net patterns and square patterns inside the concavo-convex patterns. On the belly part, there are twelve cysthuses, one of which is boldly painted smaller than others. The pot belongs to the Machang type of Majia Kiln Culture.

Provided by Qinghai Painted Ceramic Culture Society

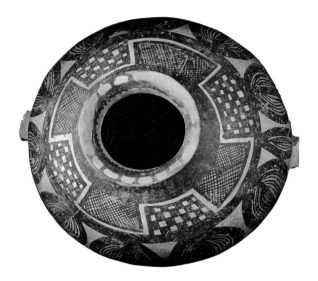

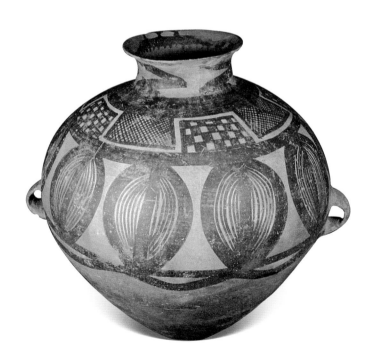

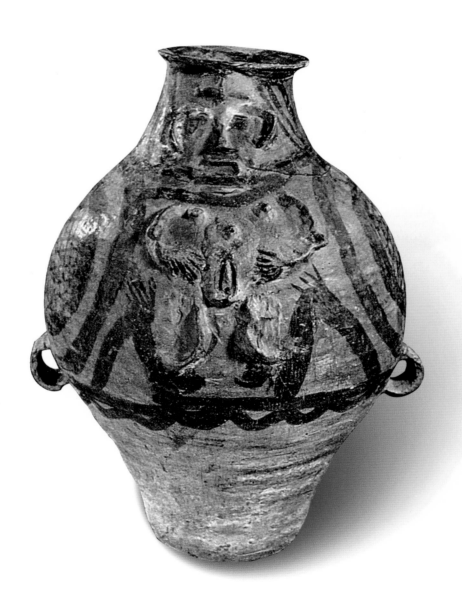

男女形裸体浮雕彩陶壶

新石器时代

细泥质褐黄陶

口径 19 厘米，高 33.4 厘米

原始宗教礼器。壶体上部施红色陶衣，于壶颈部开始有人形浮雕，头部五官俱全，长眼，大嘴，高鼻梁，大耳垂，双臂捧如孕妇的腹部，胸部裸露，乳房和乳头似曾有过哺乳史之妇女，下身兼有男、女性器官，下肢纤细。属马家窑文化马厂类型。青海省乐都县柳湾村出土。

中国国家博物馆藏

Ceramic Relief Pot with Patterns of Naked Male and Females

The Neolithic Age

Brown Argillaceous Ceramic

Mouth Diameter 19 cm/ Height 33.4 cm

It is a primitive religious ritual instrument. The upper part of the pot body is coated red, and the neck part has human relieves, each with complete facial features, including long eyes, a high nose, a big mouth and big ears. Their arms are put around the belly as if they are pregnant. Their chests are bare and their breasts and nipples show that they might have done breastfeeding. Their limbs are slender and they have both male and female sex organs. The pot belongs to the Machang type of Majia Kiln Culture. It was unearthed in Liuwan Village, Ledu County, Qinghai Province.

Preserved in National Museum of China

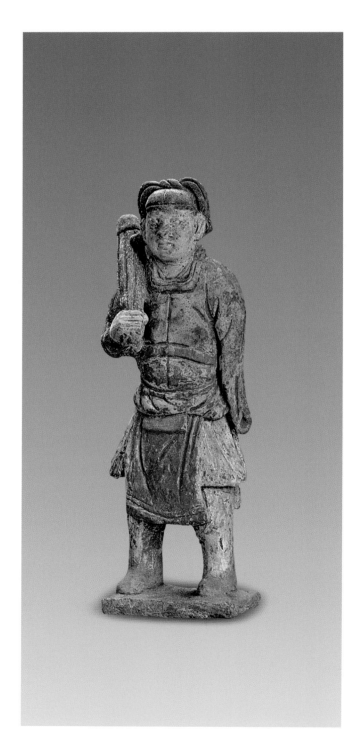

彩绘扛伞男俑

元

陶质

底座长 10.2 厘米，底座宽 7.5 厘米，高 32 厘米

Painted Male Figurine Holding an Umbrella

Yuan Dynasty

Ceramic

Bottom Length 10.2 cm/ Bottom Width 7.5 cm/

Height 32 cm

陶俑头戴黑色圆帽,帽顶打一软结垂于双耳后。高鼻大眼,络腮胡,内着右衽衣,外穿黑色方领开襟窄袖短袍,腰束革带,足蹬长靴,左臂下垂,右手握伞,扛于右肩。2007 年 5 月 14 日,河南省焦作市中站区许衡街道办事处东王封村元太医院副使靳德茂墓出土。

焦作市博物馆藏

With a black bonnet on his head, a soft knot dangling behind his ears from the bonnet, the figurine is typical of a rising nose, big eyes, and whiskers. He wears a black short open robe with narrow sleeves and a square collar over a right-fastening shirt, a leather belt around his waist, and thigh boots on his feet. With his left arm hanging down, he holds an umbrella in his right hand and rests it on his right shoulder. On May 14, 2007, the figurine was unearthed from the grave of Jin Demao, a Deputy Director of the Imperial Medical Academy in the Yuan Dynasty, at Dongwangfeng Village, Xuheng Street Community, Zhongzhan District, Jiaozuo City, Henan Province.

Preserved in Jiaozuo Museum

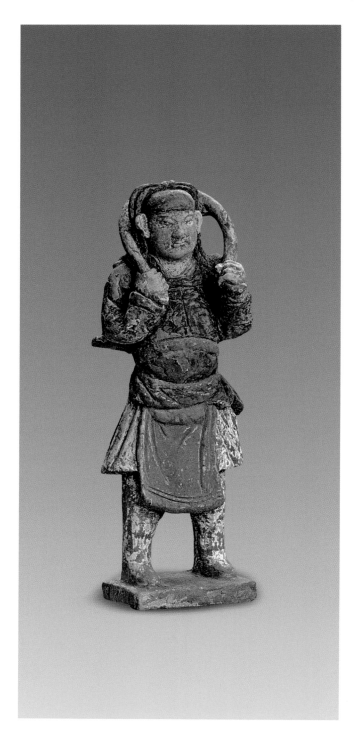

彩绘背椅男俑

元

陶质

底座长 10 厘米，底座宽 7.4 厘米，高 32.7 厘米

Painted Male Figurine Carrying a Chair

Yuan Dynasty

Ceramic

Bottom Length 10 cm/ Bottom Width 7.4 cm/

Height 32.7 cm

陶俑头戴黑色圆帽，帽顶打一软结垂于双耳后。高鼻大眼，络腮胡，内着右衽衣，外穿黑色方领开襟窄袖短袍，腰束革带，足蹬长靴，身背圈椅。2007 年 5 月 14 日，河南省焦作市中站区许衡街道办事处东王封村元太医院副使靳德茂墓出土。

焦作市博物馆藏

With a black bonnet on his head, a soft knot dangling behind his ears from the bonnet, the figurine is typical of a rising nose, big eyes, and whiskers. He wears a black short open robe with narrow sleeves and a square collar over a right-fastening shirt, a leather belt around his waist, and thigh boots on his feet. He carries a chair on his back. On May 14, 2007, the figurine was unearthed from the grave of Jin Demao, a Deputy Director of the Imperial Medical Academy in the Yuan Dynasty, at Dongwangfeng Village, Xuheng Street Community, Zhongzhan District, Jiaozuo City, Henan Province.

Preserved in Jiaozuo Museum

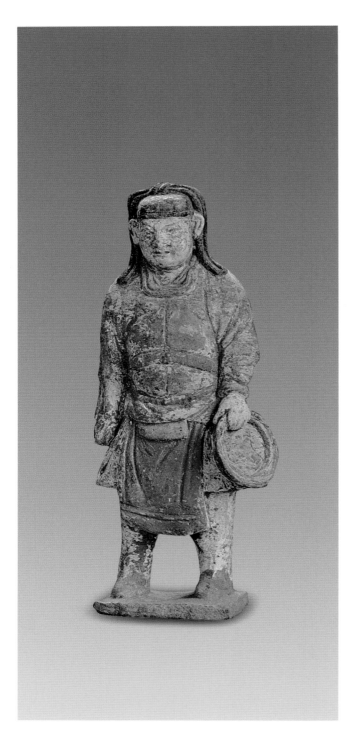

彩绘提盆男俑

元

陶质

底座长 10.2 厘米，底座宽 7.1 厘米，高 31.8 厘米

Painted Male Figurine Holding a Basin

Yuan Dynasty

Ceramic

Bottom Length 10.2 cm/ Bottom Width 7.1 cm/ Height 31.8 cm

陶俑头戴黑色圆帽，帽顶打一软结垂于双耳后。高鼻大眼，络腮胡，内着右衽衣，外穿黑色方领开襟窄袖短袍，腰束革带，足蹬长靴，左手提盆，右臂下垂。2007年5月14日，河南省焦作市中站区许衡街道办事处东王封村元太医院副使靳德茂墓出土。

焦作市博物馆藏

With a black bonnet on his head, a soft knot dangling behind his ears from the bonnet, the figurine is typical of a rising nose, big eyes, and whiskers. He wears a black short open robe with narrow sleeves and a square collar over a right-fastening shirt, a leather belt around his waist, and thigh boots on his feet. With his right arm hanging down, he holds a basin in his left hand. On May 14, 2007, the figurine was unearthed from the grave of Jin Demao, a Deputy Director of the Imperial Medical Academy in the Yuan Dynasty, at Dongwangfeng Village, Xuheng Street Community, Zhongzhan District, Jiaozuo City, Henan Province.

Preserved in Jiaozuo Museum

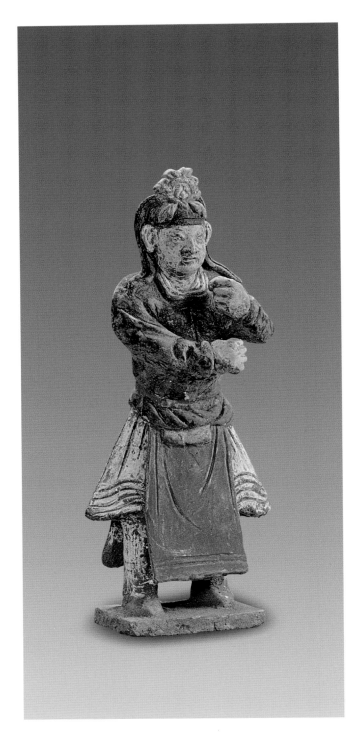

彩绘双手持物男俑

元

陶质

底座长 10.2 厘米，底座宽 8.2 厘米，高 34.3 厘米

Painted Male Figurine with Holding Hands

Yuan Dynasty

Ceramic

Bottom Length 10.2 cm/ Bottom Width 8.2 cm/

Height 34.3 cm

陶俑头戴黑色圆帽，上插华饰，帽顶打一软结垂于双耳后。高鼻大眼，络腮胡，内着右衽衣，外穿黑色方领开襟窄袖短袍，腰束革带，足蹬长靴，双手曲于胸前，做持物状。2007年5月14日，河南省焦作市中站区许衡街道办事处东王封村元太医院副使靳德茂墓出土。

焦作市博物馆藏

With a black gorgeously ornamented bonnet on his head, a soft knot dangling behind his ears from the bonnet, the figurine is typical of a rising nose, big eyes, and whiskers. He wears a black short open robe with narrow sleeves and a square collar over a right-fastening shirt, a leather belt around his waist, and thigh boots on his feet. He bends both arms in a holding gesture on his chest. On May 14, 2007, the figurine was unearthed from the grave of Jin Demao, a Deputy Director of Imperial Medical Academy in the Yuan Dynasty, at Dongwangfeng Village, Xuheng Street Community, Zhongzhan District, Jiaozuo City, Henan Province.
Preserved in Jiaozuo Museum

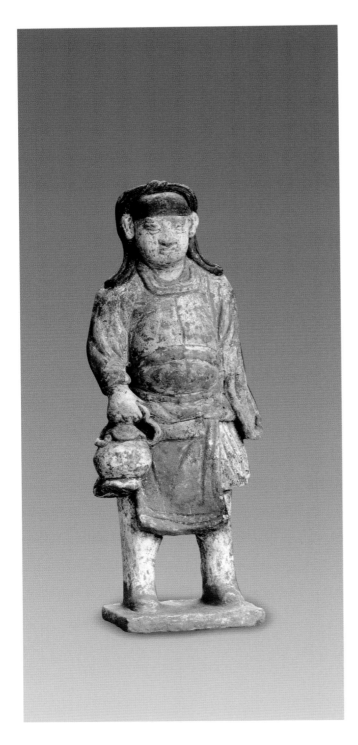

彩绘提壶男俑

元

陶质

底座长 10 厘米，底座宽 7.4 厘米，高 32.3 厘米

Painted Male Figurine Carrying a Pot

Yuan Dynasty

Ceramic

Bottom Length 10 cm/ Bottom Width 7.4 cm/

Height 32.3 cm

陶俑头戴黑色圆帽，帽顶打一软结垂于双耳后。高鼻大眼，络腮胡，内着右衽衣，外穿黑色方领开襟窄袖短袍，腰束革带，足蹬长靴，左臂窄袖长摆自然下垂，右手提壶。2007年5月14日，河南省焦作市中站区许衡街道办事处东王封村元太医院副使靳德茂墓出土。

焦作市博物馆藏

With a black bonnet on his head, a soft knot dangling behind his ears from the bonnet, the figurine is typical of a rising nose, big eyes, and whiskers. He wears a black short open robe with narrow sleeves and a square collar over a right-fastening shirt, a leather belt around his waist, and thigh boots on his feet. With his left arm hanging down naturally in the narrow sleeve, he holds a pot in his right hand. On May 14, 2007, the figurine was unearthed from the grave of Jin Demao, a Deputy Director of the Imperial Medical Academy in the Yuan Dynasty, at Dongwangfeng Village, Xuheng Street Community, Zhongzhan District, Jiaozuo City, Henan Province.

Preserved in Jiaozuo Museum

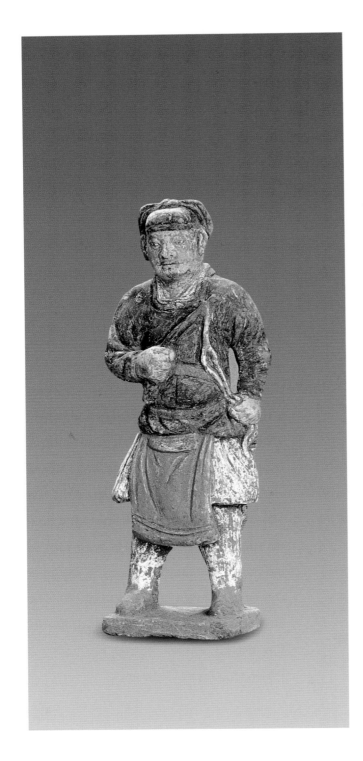

彩绘持鞭男俑

元

陶质

底座长 9.7 厘米，底座宽 7 厘米，高 31.7 厘米

Painted Male Figurine Holding a Whip

Yuan Dynasty

Ceramic

Bottom Length 9.7 cm/ Bottom Width 7 cm/

Height 31.7 cm

陶俑头戴黑色圆帽，帽顶打一软结垂于双耳后。高鼻大眼，络腮胡，内着右衽衣，外穿黑色方领开襟窄袖短袍，腰束革带，足蹬长靴，右手握鞭屈于胸前，左手持鞭梢置于腰间。2007年5月14日，河南省焦作市中站区许衡街道办事处东王封村元太医院副使靳德茂墓出土。

焦作市博物馆藏

With a black bonnet on his head, a soft knot dangling behind his ears from the bonnet, the figurine is typical of a rising nose, big eyes, and whiskers. He wears a black short open robe with narrow sleeves and a square collar over a right-fastening shirt, a leather belt around his waist, and thigh boots on his feet. He holds a whip in the right hand in front of his chest with the whip tip in the left hand on his waist. On May 14, 2007, the figurine was unearthed from the grave of Jin Demao, a Deputy Director of the Imperial Medical Academy in the Yuan Dynasty, at Dongwangfeng Village, Xuheng Street Community, Zhongzhan District, Jiaozuo City, Henan Province.

Preserved in Jiaozuo Museum

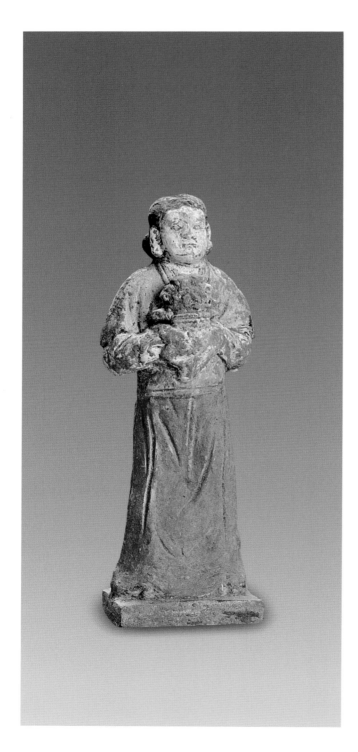

彩绘捧帽花女俑

元

陶质

底座长 9.9 厘米，底座宽 6.9 厘米，高 28.8 厘米

Colored Ceramic Woman Holding a Corsage Flower

Yuan Dynasty

Ceramic

Bottom Length 9.9 cm/ Bottom Width 6.9 cm/

Height 28.8 cm

陶俑黑髻垂于脑后。面颊丰腴，耳佩圆形耳
饰，短颈，削肩，内着白色内衣，外穿绿色
开领半臂衣，下着红裙，手捧帽花置于胸前。
2007 年 5 月 14 日，河南省焦作市中站区许
衡街道办事处东王封村元太医院副使靳德茂
墓出土。

焦作市博物馆藏

With her black hair hanging on the back of
her head and a full and round face, the colored
ceramic woman wears round earrings. She has
a short neck and slim shoulders. She wears
white underwear, green half-armed clothes with
an open collar and a red skirt, holding a corsage
flower in her hands in front of her breast. The
figurine was unearthed at Jin Demao's tomb
in Dongwangfeng Village, Xuheng Street
Community, Zhongzhan District, Jiaozuo City,
Henan Province on May 14, 2007. Jin Demao
was an assistant administrative officer of the
Imperial Academy of Medicine in the Yuan
Dynasty.

Preserved in Jiaozuo Museum

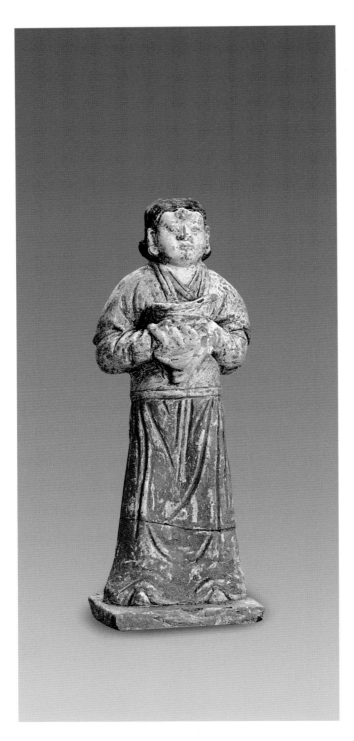

彩绘捧匜女俑

元

陶质

底座长 10.1 厘米，底座宽 7.4 厘米，高 28.3 厘米

Colored Ceramic Woman Holding a Handwashing Vessel Yi

Yuan Dynasty

Ceramic

Bottom Length10.1 cm/ Bottom Width 7.4 cm/ Height 28.3 cm

陶俑黑髻垂于脑后。面颊丰腴，耳佩圆形耳饰，短颈，削肩，内着白色内衣，外穿绿色开领半臂衣，下着红裙，双手捧匜置于胸前。2007 年 5 月 14 日，河南省焦作市中站区许衡街道办事处东王封村元太医院副使靳德茂墓出土。

焦作市博物馆藏

With her black hair hanging on the back of her head and a full and round face, the colored ceramic woman wears round earrings. She has a short neck and slim shoulders. She wears white underwear, green half-armed clothes with an open collar and a red skirt, holding a handwashing vessel Yi in her hands in front of her breast. The figurine was unearthed at Jin Demao's tomb in Dongwangfeng Village, Xuheng Street Community, Zhongzhan District, Jiaozuo City, Henan Province on May 14, 2007. Jin Demao was an assistant administrative officer of the Imperial Academy of Medicine in the Yuan Dynasty.

Preserved in Jiaozuo Museum

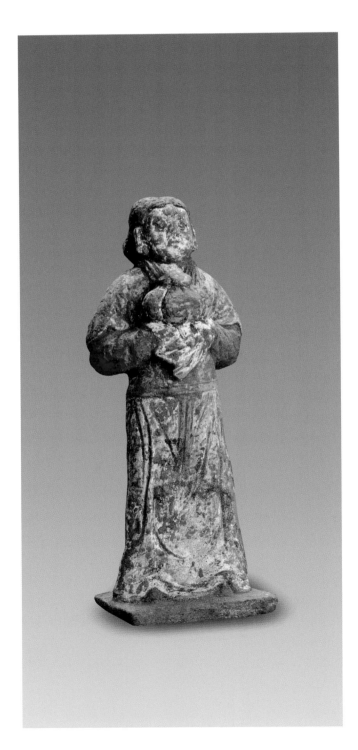

彩绘捧酒坛女俑

元

陶质

底座长 10 厘米，底座宽 8 厘米，高 28 厘米

Colored Ceramic Woman Holding a Wine Jar

Yuan Dynasty

Ceramic

Bottom Length 10 cm/ Bottom Width 8 cm/

Height 28 cm

陶俑黑髻垂于脑后。面颊丰腴，耳佩圆形耳饰，短颈，削肩，内着白色内衣，外穿绿色开领半臂衣，下着红裙，双手捧酒坛置于胸前。2007 年 5 月 14 日，河南省焦作市中站区许衡街道办事处东王封村元太医院副使靳德茂墓出土。

焦作市博物馆藏

With her black hair hanging on the back of her head and a full and round face, the colored ceramic woman wears round earrings. She has a short neck and slim shoulders. She wears white underwear, green half-armed clothes with an open collar and a red skirt, holding a wine jar in her arms in front of her breast. The figurine was unearthed at Jin Demao's tomb in Dongwangfeng Village, Xuheng Street Community, Zhongzhan District, Jiaozuo City, Henan Province on May 14, 2007. Jin Demao was an assistant administrative officer of the Imperial Academy of Medicine in the Yuan Dynasty.

Preserved in Jiaozuo Museum

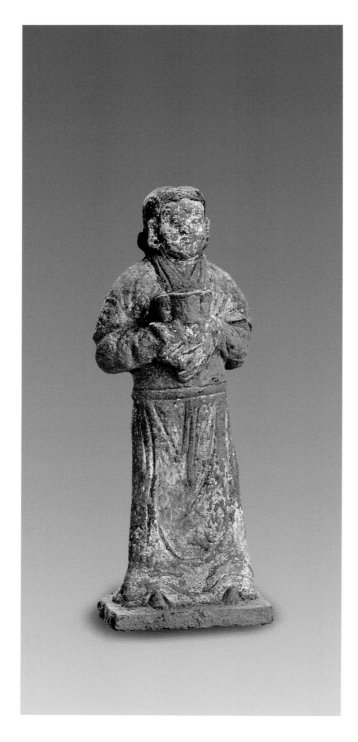

彩绘捧杯女俑

元

陶质

底座长 10.1 厘米，底座宽 7.4 厘米，高 28.3 厘米

Colored Ceramic Woman Holding a Cup

Yuan Dynasty

Ceramic

Bottom Length 10.1 cm/ Bottom Width 7.4 cm/

Height 28.3 cm

陶俑黑髻垂于脑后。面颊丰腴，耳佩圆形耳饰，短颈削肩，内着白色内衣，外穿绿色开领半臂衣，下着红裙，双手捧杯置于胸前。2007年5月14日，河南省焦作市中站区许衡街道办事处东王封村元太医院副使靳德茂墓出土。

焦作市博物馆藏

With her black hair hanging on the back of her head and a full and round face, the colored ceramic woman wears round earrings. She has a short neck and slim shoulders. She wears white underwear, green half-armed clothes with an open collar and a red skirt, holding a cup in her arms in front of her breast. The figurine was unearthed at Jin Demao's tomb in Dongwangfeng Village, Xuheng Street Community, Zhongzhan District, Jiaozuo City, Henan Province on May 14, 2007. Jin Demao was an assistant administrative officer of the Imperial Academy of Medicine in the Yuan Dynasty.

Preserved in Jiaozuo Museum

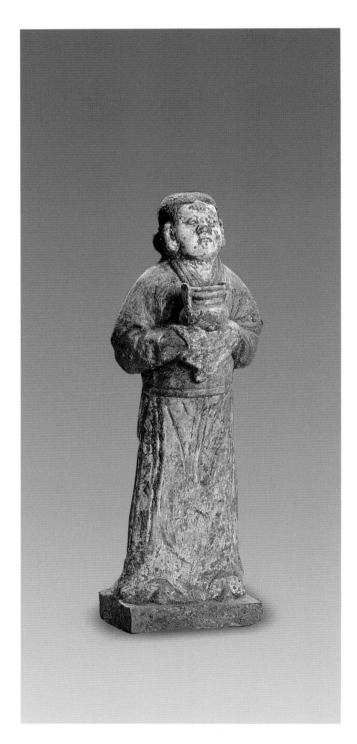

彩绘捧炉女俑

元

陶质

底座长 10.1 厘米，底座宽 7.4 厘米，高 28.3 厘米

Colored Ceramic Woman Holding a Stove

Yuan Dynasty

Ceramic

Bottom Length 10.1 cm/ Bottom Width 7.4 cm/ Height 28.3 cm

陶俑黑髻垂于脑后。面颊丰腴，耳佩圆形耳饰，短颈削肩，内着白色内衣，外穿绿色开领半臂衣，下着红裙，双手捧炉置于胸前。2007 年 5 月 14 日，河南省焦作市中站区许衡街道办事处东王封村元太医院副使靳德茂墓出土。

焦作市博物馆藏

With her black hair hanging on the back of her head and a full and round face, the colored ceramic woman wears round earrings. She has a short neck and slim shoulders. She wears white underwear, green half-armed clothes with an open collar and a red skirt, holding a stove in her arms in front of her breast. The figurine was unearthed at Jin Demao's tomb in Dongwangfeng Village, Xuheng Street Community, Zhongzhan District, Jiaozuo City, Henan Province on May 14, 2007. Jin Demao was an assistant administrative officer of the Imperial Academy of Medicine in the Yuan Dynasty.

Preserved in Jiaozuo Museum

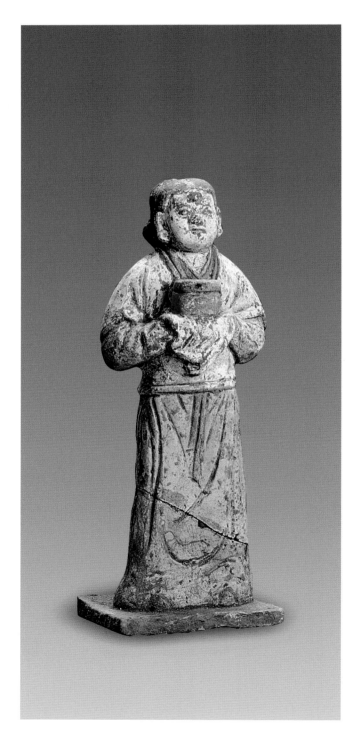

彩绘捧温酒壶女俑

元

陶质

底座长 10.3 厘米，底座宽 8 厘米，高 28 厘米

Colored Ceramic Woman Holding a Warming Wine Pot

Yuan Dynasty

Ceramic

Bottom Length 10.3 cm/ Bottom Width 8 cm/

Height 28 cm

陶俑黑髻垂于脑后。面颊丰腴，耳佩圆形耳
饰，短颈削肩，内着白色内衣，外穿绿色开
领半臂衣，下着红裙，双手捧温酒壶置于胸
前。2007 年 5 月 14 日，河南省焦作市中站
区许衡街道办事处东王封村元太医院副使靳
德茂墓出土。

焦作市博物馆藏

With her black hair hanging on the back of
her head and a full and round face, the colored
ceramic woman wears round earrings. She has a
short neck and slim shoulders. She wears white
underwear, green half-armed clothes with an
open collar and a red skirt, holding a warming
wine pot in her arms in front of her breast.
The figurine was unearthed at Jin Demao's
tomb in Dongwangfeng Village, Xuheng Street
Community, Zhongzhan District, Jiaozuo City,
Henan Province on May 14, 2007. Jin Demao
was an assistant administrative officer of the
Imperial Academy of Medicine in the Yuan
Dynasty.

Preserved in Jiaozuo Museum

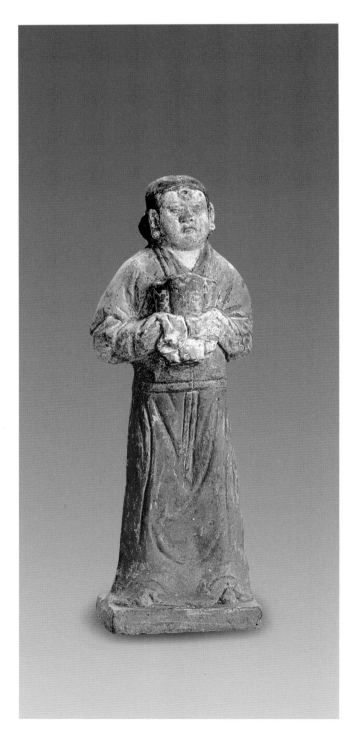

彩绘捧书卷女俑

元

陶质

底座长 9.5 厘米，底座宽 6.3 厘米，高 28 厘米

Colored Ceramic Woman Holding a Book

Yuan Dynasty

Ceramic

Bottom Length 9.5 cm/ Bottom Width 6.3 cm/ Height 28 cm

陶俑黑髻垂于脑后。面颊丰腴，耳佩圆形耳饰，短颈削肩，内着白色内衣，外穿绿色开领半臂衣，下着红裙，双手捧书置于胸前。2007 年 5 月 14 日，河南省焦作市中站区许衡街道办事处东王封村元太医院副使靳德茂墓出土。

焦作市博物馆藏

With her black hair hanging on the back of her head and a full and round face, the colored ceramic woman wears round earrings. She has a short neck and slim shoulders. She wears white underwear, green half-armed clothes with an open collar and a red skirt, holding a book in her hands in front of her breast. The figurine was unearthed at Jin Demao's tomb in Dongwangfeng Village, Xuheng Street Community, Zhongzhan District, Jiaozuo City, Henan Province on May 14, 2007. Jin Demao was an assistant administrative officer of the Imperial Academy of Medicine in the Yuan Dynasty.

Preserved in Jiaozuo Museum

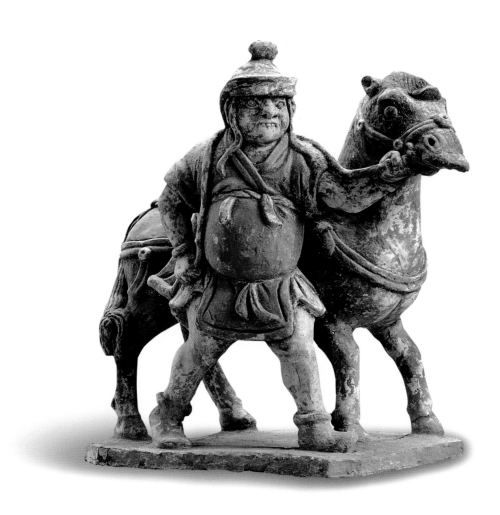

彩绘蒙古人驭马俑

元

陶质

底座长 23 厘米，底座宽 16.8 厘米，俑高 29.3 厘米，马高 28.4 厘米

陶俑为蒙古族人形象，头戴无檐宝珠顶软盔，立于马右侧，双手执缰绳。2007 年 5 月 14 日，河南省焦作市中站区许衡街道办事处东王封村元太医院副使靳德茂墓出土。

焦作市博物馆藏

Colored Ceramic Mongolian Riding a Horse

Yuan Dynasty

Ceramic

Bottom Length 23 cm/ Bottom Width 16.8 cm/ Total Height 29.3 cm/ Horse Height 28.4 cm

The colored ceramic Mongolian standing on the right side of the horse wears a soft helmet without brims, with his hands holding the reins. The figurine was unearthed at Jin Demao's tomb in Dongwangfeng Village, Xuheng Street Community, Zhongzhan District, Jiaozuo City, Henan Province on May 14, 2007. Jin Demao was an assistant administrative officer of the Imperial Academy of Medicine in the Yuan Dynasty.

Preserved in Jiaozuo Museum

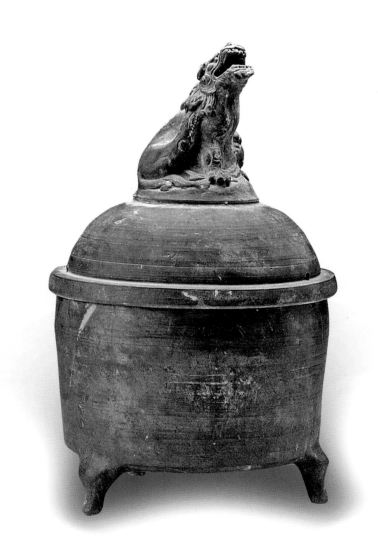

奁盒

元

陶质

直径 20 厘米，高 34 厘米

Ceramic Cosmetic Box

Yuan Dynasty

Ceramic

Diameter 20 cm/ Height 34 cm

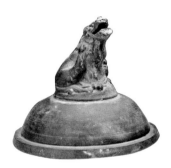

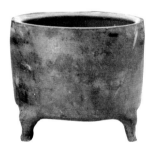

轮制。子母口，身呈直腹微向下斜收，平底，三足。仰头蹲狮形盖钮，有出香口。陕西省西安市东郊鑫元小区出土。

陕西省考古研究院藏

The wheel-made cosmetic box has a snap–lid, a flat bottom and three feet. It has a straight abdomen sloping slightly downward, a lid button in the shape of a squatting lion and an opening from which incense comes out. The box was unearthed in Xinyuan Residential Quarters in the eastern suburbs of Xi'an, Shaanxi Province.

Preserved in Shaanxi Provincial Institute of Archaeology

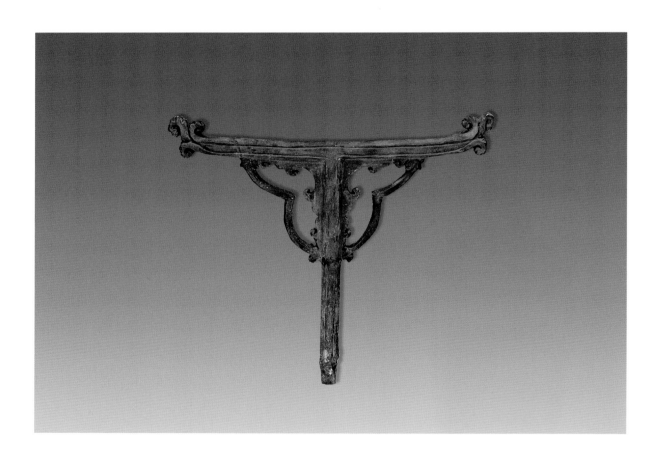

巾架

元

陶质

最宽 43 厘米，厚 2.5 厘米，最高 43 厘米

Towel Rack

Yuan Dynasty

Ceramic

Maximum Width 43 cm/ Thickness 2.5 cm/ Maximum Height 43 cm

仿木制家具。"丁"字状，搭脑两端出头，呈云头状。中央置立杆，柱头两侧有花牙子，直抵搭脑。搭脑与立柱之间两边有枨，整体呈葫芦形。1976 年，山西省大同市城东曹夫楼北崔莹李氏墓出土。

大同市博物馆藏

The T-shaped towel rack is a piece of ceramic furniture in the color of wood. There is an upright pole in the middle with serrated edge on both sides of the top. There are supporting branches between the upright pole and the rods, which makes it look like a gourd. The rack was unearthed in Mr. Li's tomb at Cuiying, north of Caofu Pavilion, east of Datong City, Shanxi Province in 1976.

Preserved in Datong Museum

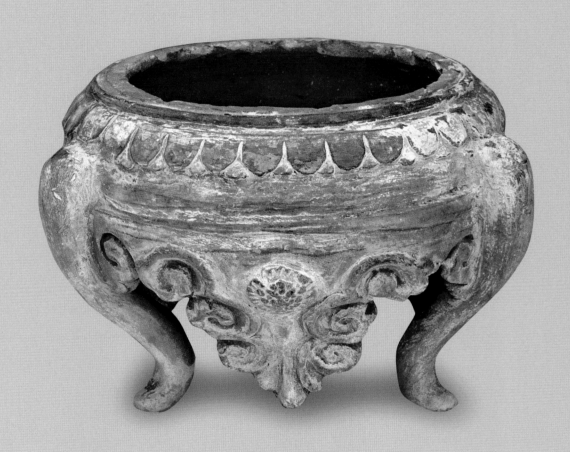

火盆架

元

陶质

口径 15 厘米，最大径 21.5 厘米，高 14.5 厘米

火盆架由罗汉腿、下衬、座圈等组成。1976 年，
山西省大同市城东曹夫楼北崔莹李氏墓出土。

大同市博物馆藏

Fire Basket Rack

Yuan Dynasty

Ceramic

Mouth Diameter 15 cm/ Maximum Diameter
21.5 cm/ Height 14.5 cm

The fire basket rack consists of arhat legs, lower
lining and the seat ring. It was unearthed in Mr.
Li's tomb at Cuiying, north of Caofu Pavilion,
east of Datong City, Shanxi Province in 1976.

Preserved in Datong Museum

塔式堆贴塑群佛跂士陶魂坛

唐

陶质

腹径 26.5 厘米，底径 14 厘米，高 39 厘米

腹上部堆塑佛像，圈足，平底。带盖，宝塔钮，盖、腹各堆塑两圈水波纹，足部堆塑一圈水波纹。仫佬族葬具。

罗城仫佬族博物馆藏

Tower Ceramic Ghost Jar Pasted with Clay Buddhas

Tang Dynasty

Ceramic

Belly Diameter 26.5 cm/ Bottom Diameter 14 cm/ Height 39 cm

The jar has a belly on the upper of which are pasted Buddha statues, as well as a round foot, a flat Bottom and a cover with a tower knot. Two rings of wave patterns are pasted on the cover and the belly, and one ring of wave patterns on the foot. It was used at Mulao's burials.

Preserved in Luocheng Mulao Museum

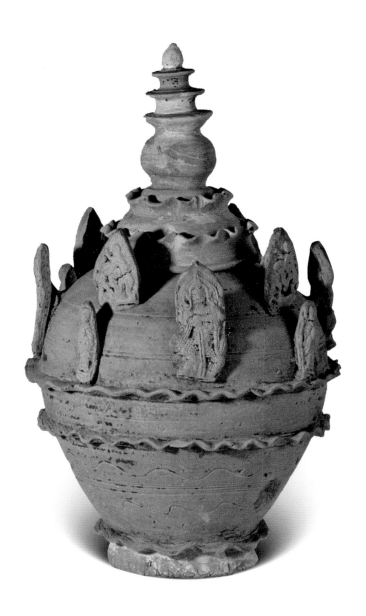

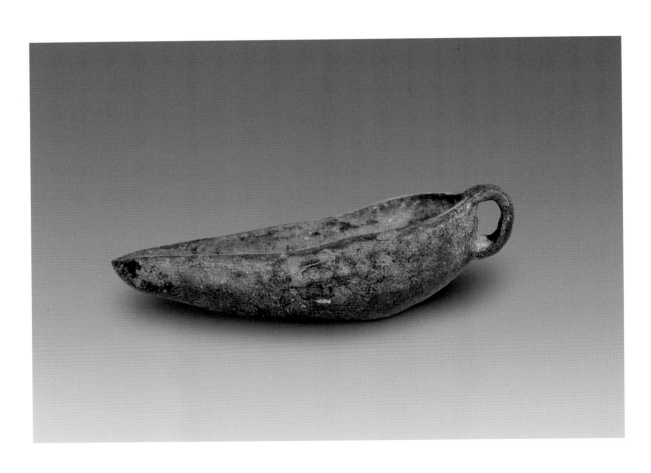

陶质船形油灯

19 世纪初

陶质

长 29 厘米，宽 14.5 厘米，高 9 厘米

Boat-shaped Ceramic Oil Lamp

Early 19th Century

Ceramic

Length 29 cm/ Width 14.5 cm/ Heigh 9 cm

船形，若一叶扁舟，灯口尖而低矮，灯身渐高、渐深、渐阔，与灯口相对有桥形把。此灯是照明用的工具。

西藏博物馆藏

The rowboat-shaped lamp has a sharp, short, and shallow mouth, and an increasingly taller, deeper and wider body. Opposite to the mouth is fixed an arched handle. It was used for lighting. Preserved in Tibet Museum

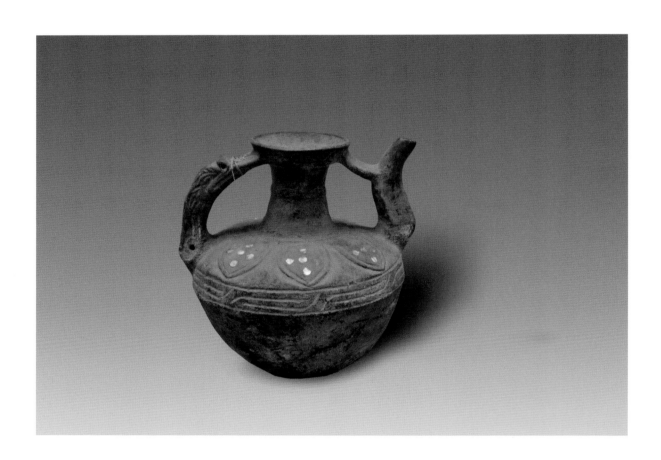

酒壶

民国时期

陶质

腹径 20 厘米，高 26 厘米

Wine Pot

Republican Period

Ceramic

Belly Diameter 20 cm/ Height 26 cm

盘口，鼓腹，平底，有流和把，腹部有旋纹，

肩部有花瓣纹，上嵌白色石块，是藏族用品。

由民间征集。

成都中医药大学中医药传统文化博物馆藏

The pot has a plate-like mouth, a protruding belly, a flat bottom, a spout and a handle. On the belly spiral lines are engraved. The pot shoulder is decorated with petals inlaid with opals. This piece of Tibetan household ware was collected from a private owner.

Preserved in Museum of Traditional Chinese Medicine Culture, Chengdu University of Traditional Chinese Medicine

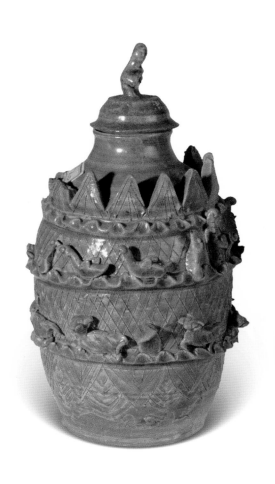
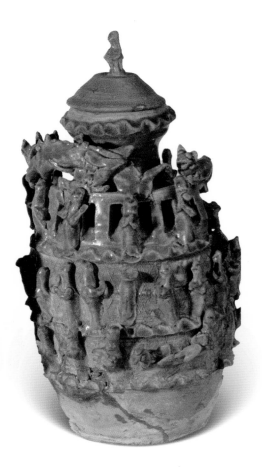

青瓷堆塑人龙虎魂瓶（一对）

北宋

瓷质

左：腹径 17 厘米，底径 11 厘米，高 26 厘米

右：腹径 18.2 厘米，底径 12.1 厘米，高 27 厘米

魂瓶，又称"谷仓罐"或"堆塑罐"。瓶为平底，堆塑人物、飞鸟、走兽等装饰图案。这是为了祭奠死者、超度亡灵而专门烧制的随葬明器。仫佬族葬具。罗城第二水厂建筑工地出土。

罗城仫佬族博物馆藏

Celadon Ghost Vase Couple Pasted with Humans, Dragons, and Tigers

Northern Song Dynasty

Porcelain

Left: Belly Diameter 17 cm/ Bottom Diameter 11 cm/ Height 26 cm

Right: Belly Diameter 18.2 cm/ Bottom Diameter 12.1 cm/ Height 27 cm

Ghost vase is also referred as "Grain Jar" or "Pasted Jar". The two jars are flatly Bottomd and decoratively pasted with patterns of humans, birds and beasts. They were specially made as funerary objects buried together with Mulao's deceased. The vase was unearthed at the construction site of No. 2 Water Plant, Luocheng Mulao Autonomous County.

Preserved in Luocheng Mulao Museum

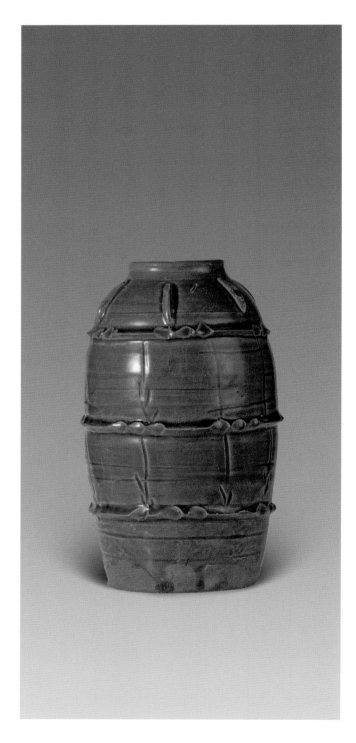

青瓷竹节式魂瓶

北宋

瓷质

口径6.8厘米，腹径12.8厘米，底径8.4厘米，
高 22.5 厘米

Bamboo-styled Celadon Ghost Vase

Northern Song Dynasty

Porcelain

Mouth Diameter 6.8 cm/ Belly Diameter 12.8 cm/

Bottom Diameter 8.4 cm/ Height 22.5 cm

魂瓶，又称"谷仓罐"或"堆塑罐"。瓶为平底，堆塑竹节纹。这是为了祭奠死者、超度亡灵而专门烧制的随葬明器。仫佬族葬具。罗城龙岸镇建筑工地出土。

罗城仫佬族博物馆藏

Ghost vase is also referred as "Grain Jar" or "Pasted Jar". This jar is flatly Bottomd and decoratively pasted with bamboo patterns. It was specially made as funerary object buried together with Mulao's deceased. It was unearthed at the construction site in Long'an Town, Luocheng Mulao Autonomous County. Preserved in Luocheng Mulao Museum

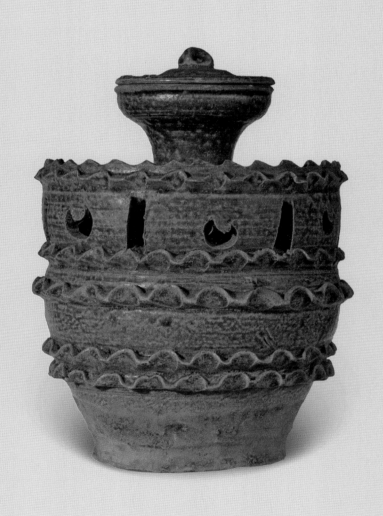

青瓷盘口带盖谷仓罐

北宋

瓷质

腹径 18.5 厘米，底径 13.2 厘米，高 28 厘米

盘口，束颈，平底，堆塑水波纹。这是为了祭奠死者、超度亡灵而专门烧制的随葬明器。仫佬族葬具。罗城东门镇章罗村出土。

罗城仫佬族博物馆藏

Covered Wide-mouthed Celadon Ghost Jar

Northern Song Dynasty

Porcelain

Belly Diameter 18.5cm/ Bottom Diameter 13.2 cm/ Height 28cm

The jar has a wide mouth, a convergent neck, and a flat Bottom pasted with wave patterns. It was specially made as funerary object for Mulao's deceased. It was unearthed at Zhangluo Village, Dongmen Town, Luocheng Mulao Autonomous County.

Preserved in Luocheng Mulao Museum

青瓷带盖圈纹魂坛

北宋

瓷质

口径 8 厘米，腹径 18 厘米，底径 10.5 厘米，
高 20 厘米

侈口，束颈，斜肩，鼓腹，平底。带盖。仡佬
族葬具。罗城小长安镇崖宜屯坡地出土。

罗城仡佬族博物馆藏

Covered Celadon Ghost Jar with Cirrus Patterns

Northern Song Dynasty

Porcelain

Mouth Diameter 8 cm/ Belly Diameter 18 cm/
Bottom Diameter 10.5 cm/ Height 20 cm

The jar has a wide mouth, a convergent neck,
a sloping shoulder, a protruding belly, a flat
Bottom, and a cover. It was used at Mulao's
burials. It was unearthed at a slope at Yayitun
Village in Xiaochang'an Town, Luocheng Mulao
Autonomous County.

Preserved in Luocheng Mulao Museum

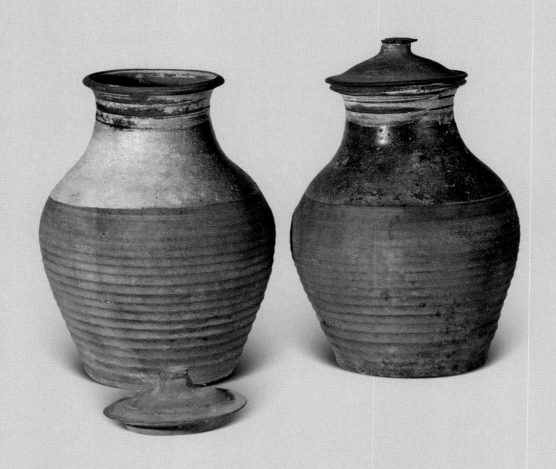

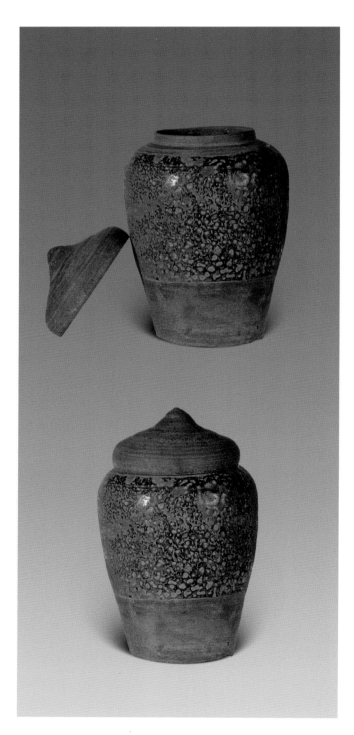

青瓷带盖丰肩魂坛

北宋

瓷质

口径6.8厘米，肩颈15.6厘米，底径7.4厘米，
高20厘米

Covered Celadon Ghost Jar with a Broad Shoulder

Northern Song Dynasty

Porcelain

Mouth Diameter 6.8 cm/ Shoulder Diameter
15.6 cm/ Bottom Diameter 7.4 cm/ Height 20 cm

子母口，丰肩，鼓腹，平底。带盖。仫佬族葬具。
罗城小长安镇双河村出土。

罗城仫佬族博物馆藏

The jar has a synthesized set of mouths, a broad
shoulder, a protruding belly, a flat Bottom and
a cover. It was used at Mulao's burials. It was
unearthed at Shuanghe Village, Xiaochang'an
Town, Luocheng Mulao Autonomous County.
Preserved in Luocheng Mulao Museum

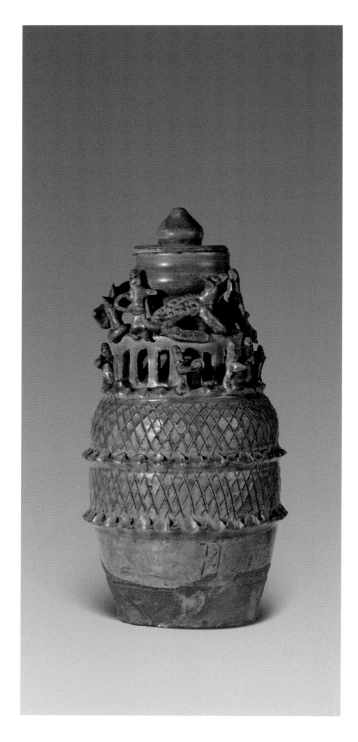

青瓷捏塑乐俑动物刻画网纹魂瓶

南宋

瓷质

口径 7 厘米，腹径 16.8 厘米，底径 11.5 厘米，
高 30.5 厘米

Celadon Ghost Vase with Kneaded Patterns of Musician Figurines and Beasts and Carved Net Patterns

Southern Song Dynasty

Porcelain

Mouth Diameter 7 cm/ Belly Diameter 16.8 cm/

Bottom Diameter 11.5 cm/ Height 30.5 cm

魂瓶，又称"谷仓罐"或"堆塑罐"。瓶为平底，捏塑乐俑动物纹。腹部捏塑水波纹，刻画网纹。这是为了祭奠死者、超度亡灵而专门烧制的仡佬族随葬明器。罗城黄金镇古岭坪屯坡出土。

罗城仡佬族博物馆藏

Ghost vase is also referred as "Grain Jar" or "Pasted Jar". This flat-Bottomd vase is decorated with kneaded musician figurines and beasts. On the belly are also kneaded wave patterns and carved net patterns. It was specially made as funerary object buried together with Mulao's deceased. The vase was unearthed at a slope at Gulingping Village, Huangjin Town, Luocheng Mulao Autonomous County.

Preserved in Luocheng Mulao Museum

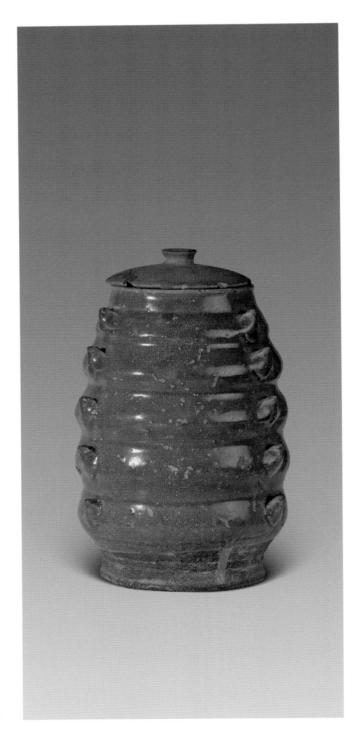

青瓷蚕蛹形魂瓶

南宋

瓷质

口径9厘米，腹径15厘米，底径10.2厘米，

高24厘米

Silkworm-shaped Celadon Ghost Vase

Southern Song Dynasty

Porcelain

Mouth Diameter 9 cm/ Belly Diameter 15 cm/

Bottom Diameter 10.2 cm/ Height 24 cm

魂瓶，又称"谷仓罐"或"堆塑罐"。这是为了祭奠死者、超度亡灵而专门烧制的仡佬族随葬明器。罗城东门镇旧县署建筑工地出土。

罗城仡佬族博物馆藏

Ghost vase is also referred as "Grain Jar" or "Pasted Jar". It was specially made as funerary object buried together with Mulao's deceased. It was unearthed at the construction site at the former magistrates' office, Dongmen Town, Luocheng Mulao Autonomous County.

Preserved in Luocheng Mulao Museum

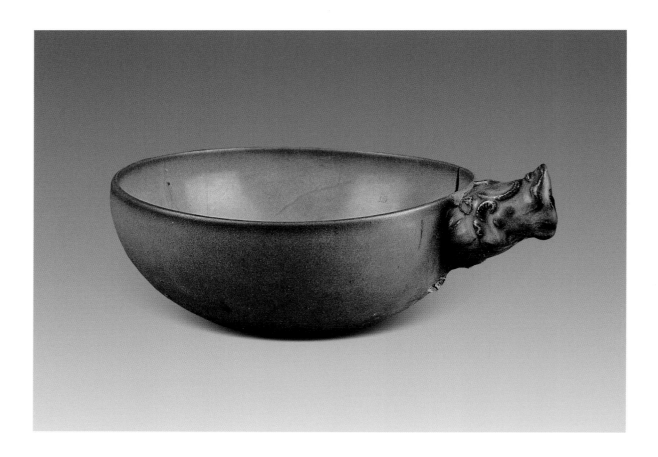

钧窑龙首匜

元

瓷质

宽 18.6 厘米，高 8 厘米

Jun Kiln Dragon Head-shaped Washing Vessel Yi

Yuan Dynasty

Porcelain

Width 18.6 cm/ Height 8 cm

圆口，深腹，平底，杯柄塑龙首流，中有流孔。施天蓝釉，口沿施米黄釉，釉面细密，胎质细腻。此匜圆浑粗犷，造型别致，颇具匠心。用于沃盥之礼，为客人洗手所用。此为元代蒙古族典型的盥洗时舀水用器具。河北省定兴县河内村张弘范家族6号墓出土。

定兴县文物保护管理所藏

This vessel has a round mouth, a deep belly, a flat Bottom and a spout shaped as a dragon head. The smooth body is fully glazed sky blue but cream on the mouth. The vessel, vigorous and pure, is shaped uniquely and exquisitely. As a typical washing ware of the Mongolians in Yuan Dynasty, it was gravely used to spout water for their guests' hands. The vessel was unearthed from Tomb No. 6 of Zhang Hongfan's family at Henei Village, Dingxing County, Hebei Province. Preserved in Dingxing Cultural Relics Management Institute

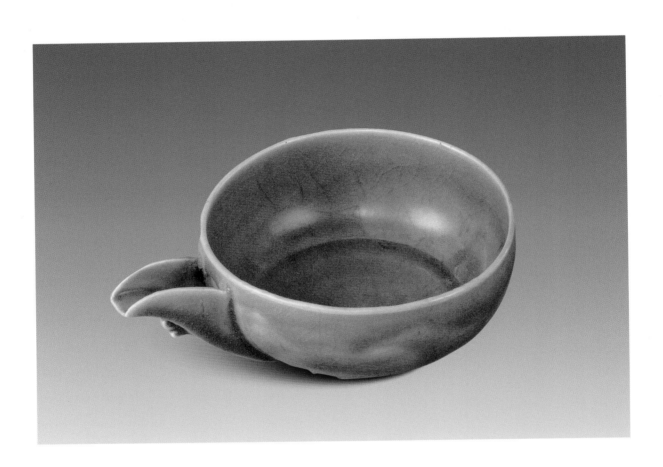

龙泉窑青釉瓷匜

元

瓷质

口径 14.2 厘米，足径 8.4 厘米，高 6.3 厘米

Longquan Kiln Celadon Vessel Yi

Yuan Dynasty

Porcelain

Mouth Diameter 14.2 cm/ Foot Diameter 8.4 cm/ Height 6.3 cm

敞口，弧形腹，平底，口沿一侧有流，流下有一卷云状耳。用于沃盥之礼，为客人洗手所用。为元代蒙古族典型的盥洗时用具。甘肃省漳县汪世显家族墓出土。

甘肃省博物馆藏

The open vessel has an arch belly and a flat Bottom. From the mouth leads a spout under which lies a handle in the shape of rolling clouds. As a typical washing ware of the Mongolians in the Yuan Dynasty, it was gravely used to spout water for their guests' hands. It was unearthed from the tomb of Wang Shixian's family in Zhang County, Gansu Province.

Preserved in Gansu Provincial Museum

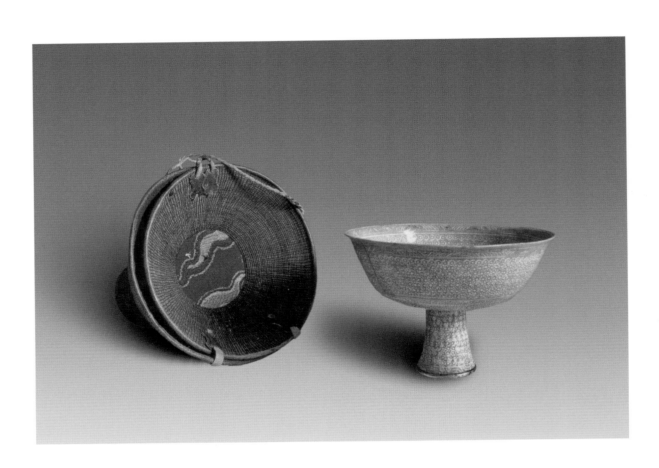

青釉菊花纹高足碗

高丽

瓷质

口径 14.7 厘米，底径 4.1 厘米，高 10.5 厘米，足高 4.8 厘米

Celadon-Glazed Stem Bowl with Chrysanthemum Decoration

Korea Dynasty

Porcelain

Mouth Diameter 14.7 cm/ Bottom Diameter 4.1 cm/ Height 10.5 cm/ Foot Height 4.8 cm

侈口，敛腹，高足外撇。青釉，菊花纹。配有制作精美的碗套。

西藏博物馆藏

The bowl is glazed with celadon over its wide an outstretching mouth, a contracting belly, and an outward high foot, and decorated with chrysanthemum patterns. It is in a complete set with an ornate cover.

Preserved in Tibet Museum

景泰蓝番莲纹僧帽碗

明

瓷质

口径 11 厘米，宽 20 厘米，底径 8 厘米，高 22.5 厘米

壶口形似僧帽，口沿上翘，前低后高，鸭嘴形流，壶盖卧于口沿内，束颈，鼓腹，平底，圈足，曲柄，具有浓郁的少数民族风格。

西藏博物馆藏

Mitre-shaped Cloisonne Bowl with Passionfrace Design

Ming Dynasty

Porcelain

Mouth Diameter 11 cm/ Width 20 cm/ Bottom Diameter 8 cm/ Height 22.5 cm

The Mouth is shaped as a miter, with a brim tilt up to the real and a duckbilled spout in the front. The cover elaborately fits into the mouth. With a convergent neck, a bulging body, a flat Bottom, and a ring foot, the bowl is strongly featured with styles of the ethnical minority.

Preserved in Tibet Museum

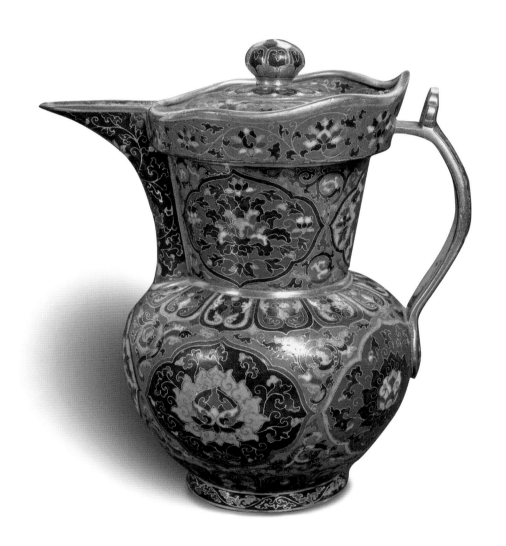

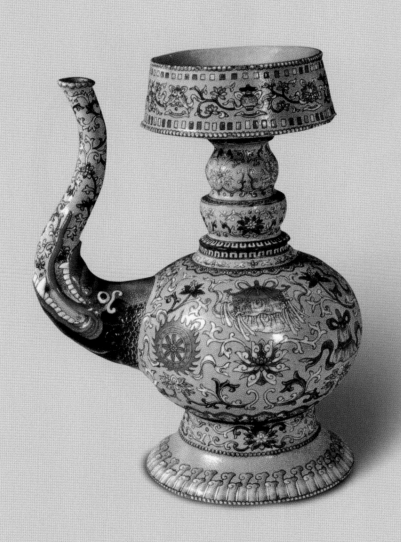

景泰蓝净水瓶

清·乾隆

瓷质

口径 7.5 厘米，底径 10 厘米，高 20 厘米

珐琅釉。兽首吐长流，葫芦颈，溜肩，鼓腹，平底，圈足外撇，具有装饰性和实用性。盛水器皿。

西藏博物馆藏

Cloisonne Water Bottle

Qianlong Period, Qing Dynasty

Porcelain

Mouth Diameter 7.5 cm/ Bottom Diameter 10 cm/
Height 20 cm

The cloisonne enameled water bottle has a long-nosed head. It is featured with a gourd-shaped neck, sloping shoulders, a bulging body, and a flat outstretched foot. It is of both ornamental and practical use.

Preserved in Tibet Museum

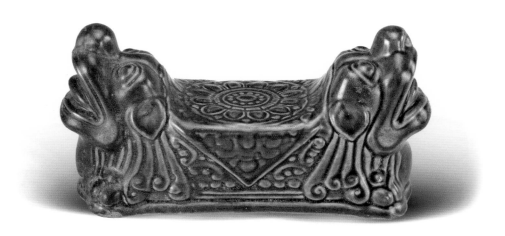

狮首瓷枕

近现代

瓷质

长 26 厘米

用于切脉和治疗颈椎病。

内蒙古医科大学蒙医药博物馆藏

Lion Head-shaped Porcelain Pillow

Modern Times

Porcelain

Length 26 cm

It was used in pulse-taking and cervical spondylosis treatment.

Preserved in Mongolian Medicine Museum of Inner Mongolia Medical University

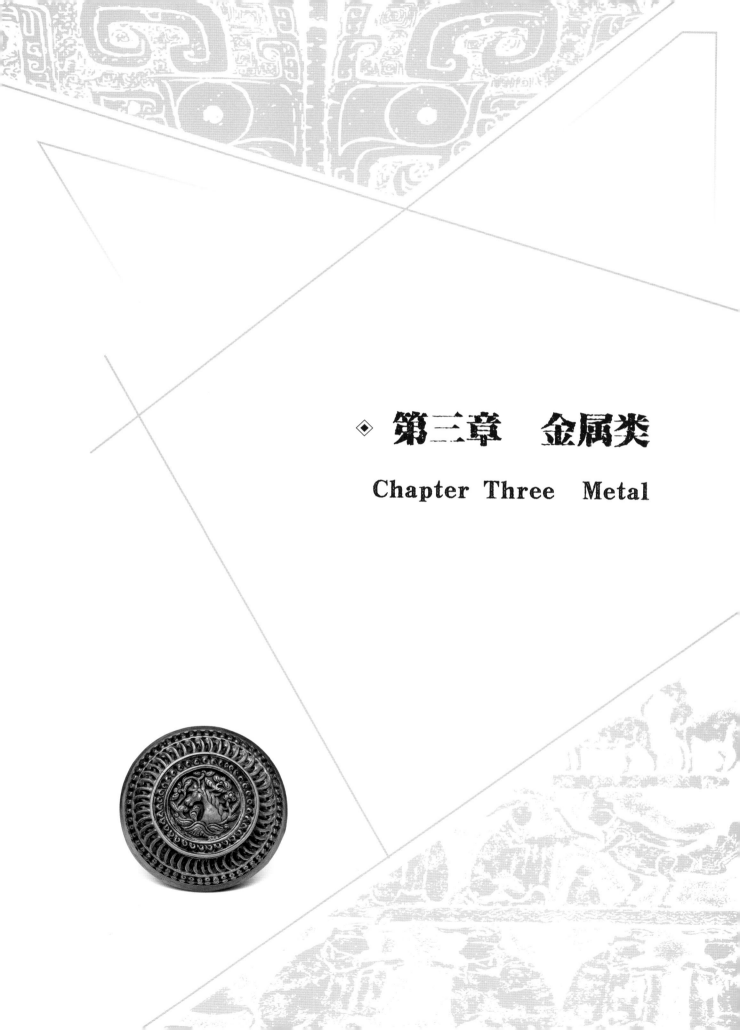

◈ 第三章 金属类

Chapter Three　Metal

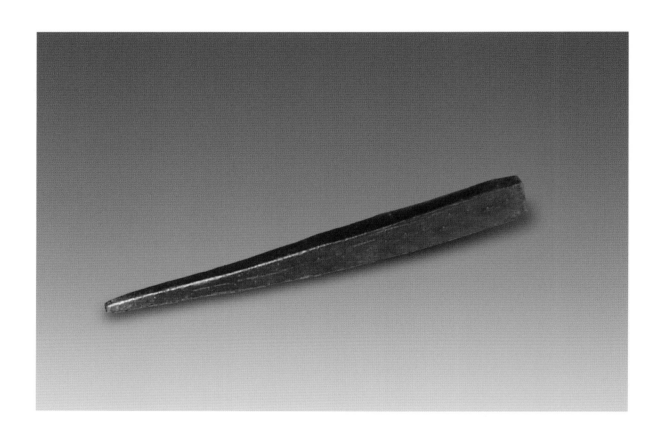

匈奴铜锥

战国时期

铜质

长 6.6 厘米，宽 0.5 厘米，重 1 克

Hunnish Copper Cone

Warring States Period

Copper

Length 6.6 cm/ Width 0.5 cm/ Weight 1 g

四棱锥状。兵器。完整无损。内蒙古自治区

成吉思汗陵征集。

陕西医史博物馆藏

This rectangular pyramid-shaped cone was a weapon. It is still in good condition. It was collected in Genghis Khan's Mausoleum, Inner Mongolia Autonomous Region.

Preserved in Shaanxi Museum of Medical History

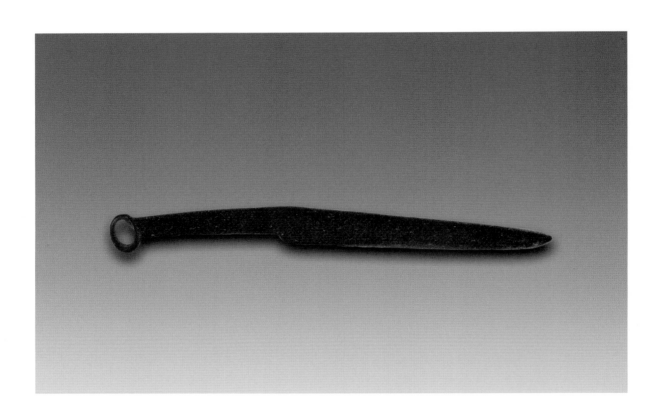

匈奴铜刀

战国时期

铜质

通长 13.6 厘米，柄长 5 厘米

Hunnish Copper Dagger

Warring States Period

Copper

Full Length 13.6 cm/ Handle Length 5 cm

匈奴生活用刀，亦用于医疗。1978 年在内蒙古伊金霍洛旗采集。

陕西医史博物馆藏

The dagger was used by the Huns either for daily or medical purpose. It was collected in Ejin Horo Banner, Inner Mongolia Autonomous Region in 1978.

Preserved in Shaanxi Museum of Medical History

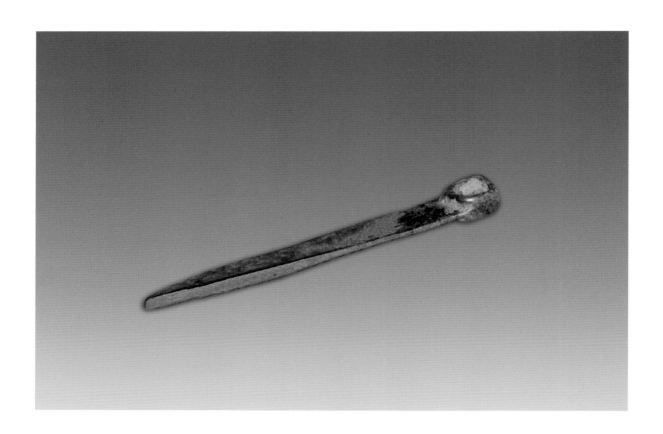

匈奴铜刀

战国时期

铜质

长 7.5 厘米，宽 1.2 厘米，重 50 克

Hunnish Copper Knife

Warring States Period

Copper

Length 7.5 cm/ Width 1.2 cm/ Weight 50 g

尖为锥形扁平，刀把有一孔。兵器。完整无损。
内蒙古自治区达拉特旗征集。

陕西医史博物馆藏

The knife takes on a cone-shaped flat tip and a
hole in the handle. Once used as a weapon, it is
still in good condition. It was collected in Dalad
Banner, Inner Mongolia Autonomous Region.
Preserved in Shaanxi Museum of Medical History

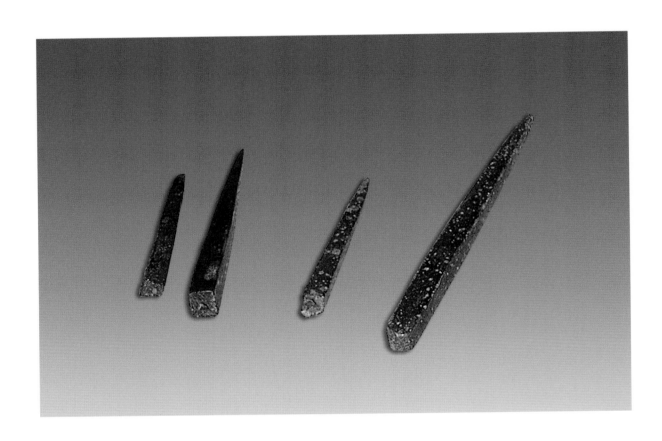

匈奴铜锥尖

汉

铜质

分别长 5 厘米、3.3 厘米、2.7 厘米、2.4 厘米，重 5 克

Hunnish Copper Cone Tips

Han Dynasty

Copper

Length 5 cm, 3.3 cm, 2.7 cm, and 2.4 cm respectively/ Weight 5 g

四棱尖状。兵器。完整无损。内蒙古自治区
东胜征集。

陕西医史博物馆藏

These rectangular pyramid-shaped cone tips
were weapons. They are still in good condition.
They were collected in Dongsheng, Inner
Mongolia Autonomous Region.
Preserved in Shaanxi Museum of Medical History

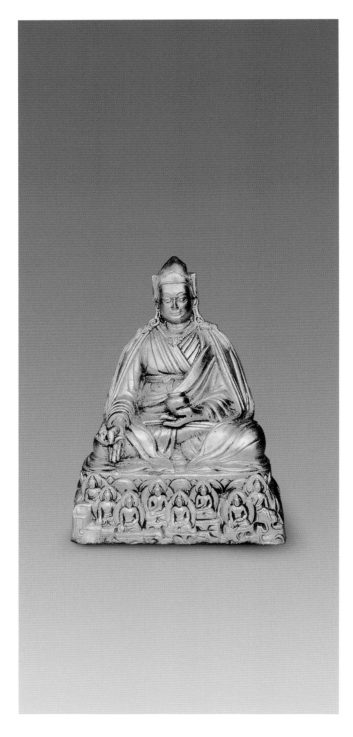

曼吉拉化身喇嘛塑像

清

镏铜

Statue of the Incarnate Lama of Manjila

Qing Dynasty

Copper-plated

曼吉拉即琉璃光佛，具有与其原型药师王佛同样的象征。塑像背部有铭文"曼吉拉解除了诸如癫痫及其他疾病等魔鬼的压迫"等，其基座前面浮塑有8个药王像。在西藏南部发现。

Manjila, Buddha of Glazed Light, shares the same status with its prototype — the Medicine Master Buddha of Vaidurya Light. The inscription on the back of the statue says "Manjila removes evil tortures of epilepsia and other diseases". The front pedestal is embossed with eight medicine masters. The statue was collected in the southern part of Tibet.

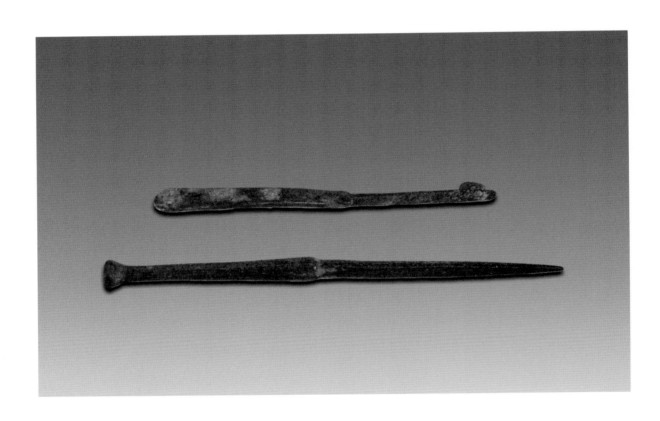

蒙医放血刀

清

铜质

长 8.3 厘米

Mongolian Doctor's Fleam

Qing Dynasty

Copper

Length 8.3 cm

蒙医放血疗法所用的刀具。1978 年在内蒙古
呼和浩特采集。

陕西医史博物馆藏

These fleams were used by Mongolian doctors
for blood-letting therapy. They were collected in
Hohhot, Inner Mongolia Autonomous Region.
Preserved in Shaanxi Museum of Medical History

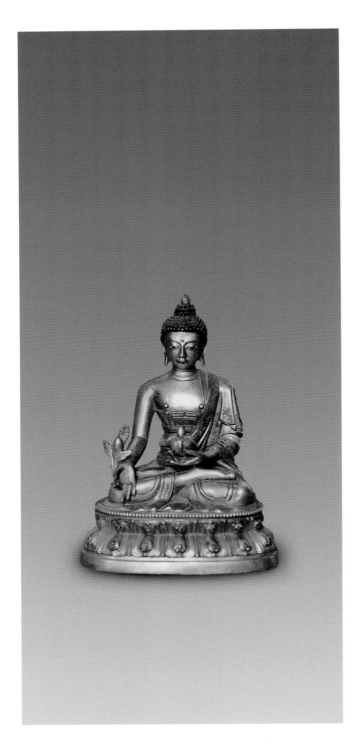

乃木其像

清

座宽 9 厘米，通高 16.5 厘米

Naimuqi Statue

Qing Dynasty

Bottom Width 9 cm/ Height 16.5 cm

塑像上为佛像，下为莲房，庄重端秀。佛像一手持草状物（柯黎子），一手捧仙桃。据专家确认为乃木其像。乃木其即汉语的净眼如来，是佛经中的药王菩萨星宿光。

陕西医史博物馆藏

The statue is a Buddha meditating on a pedestal embossed with lotus flowers. Solemnly but elegantly, the Buddha holds a herb straw in one hand, and a longevity peach in the other. Experts confirmed that the Buddha is Naimuqi, the Chinese name for Tathagata, the Medicine Master Buddha.

Preserved in Shaanxi Museum of Medical History

铜烤炉

清

铜质

长 70 厘米

用于煎药或饮食疗法。

内蒙古博物院藏

Copper Oven

Qing Dynasty

Copper

Length 70 cm

It was used to boil medicinal herbs or in the diet

therapy.

Preserved in Inner Mongolia Museum

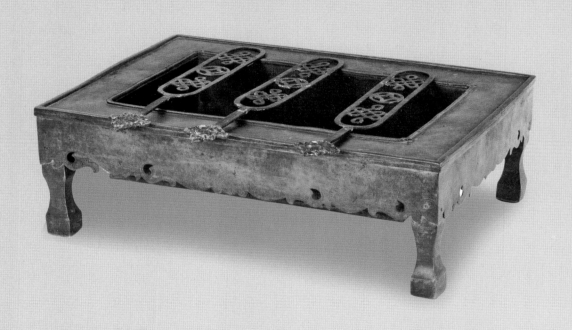

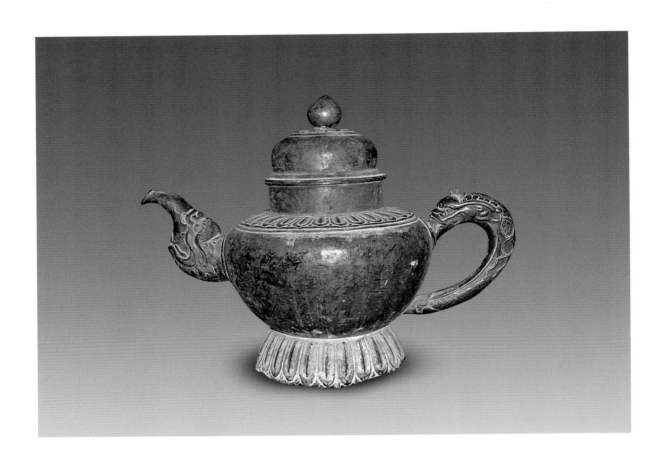

藏铜壶

清

铜质

口径 14.5 厘米，底径 28 厘米，通高 33.5 厘米，重 2200 克

Tibetan Copper Pot

Qing Dynasty

Copper

Mouth Diameter 14.5 cm/ Bottom Diameter 28 cm/ Height 33.5 cm/ Weight 2,200 g

子母口，直颈，鼓腹，龙头壶嘴，龙手把。

生活用器。基本完整。陕西省汉中市征集。

陕西医史博物馆藏

As a daily article, the pot has a synthesized set of mouths, a straight neck, a bulging body, a dragonhead-shaped spout and a dragon-shaped handle. It is in good condition. It was collected in Hanzhong City, Shaanxi Province.

Preserved in Shaanxi Museum of Medical History

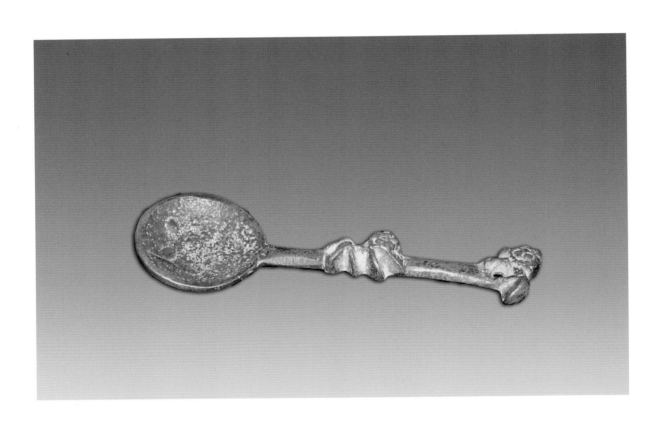

蒙医药勺

清

铜质

长 8.9 厘米，勺径 2.8 厘米，重 19 克

Mongolian Medicine Spoon

Qing Dynasty

Copper

Length 8.9 cm/ Spoon Diameter 2.8 cm/ Weight 19 g

勺头浅圆，勺把有浮雕。医药器具。完整无损。

陕西医史博物馆藏

The spoon is flat and round with an embossed handle. It was for medical use, and is still in good condition.

Preserved in Shaanxi Museum of Medical History

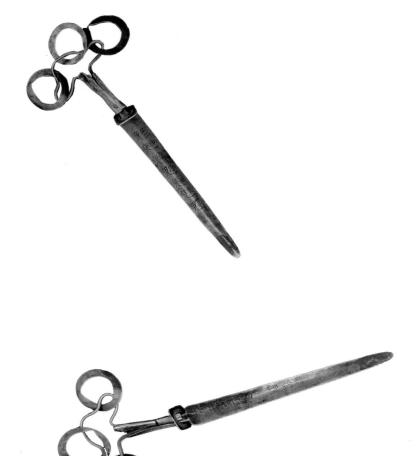

双面錾刻驱邪令铜法剑

清

铜质

长 29 厘米，最宽处 3 厘米

驱邪用具。罗城东门镇横岸村传世藏品。

吴桂文藏

Copper Magic Sword Engraved with Exorcism Spells on Both Sides

Qing Dynasty

Copper

Length 29 cm/ Maximum Width 3 cm

It was used to expel evil spirits. It is handed down as a precious heritage of Heng'an Village, Dongmen Town, Luocheng Mulao Autonomous County.

Collected by Wu Guiwen

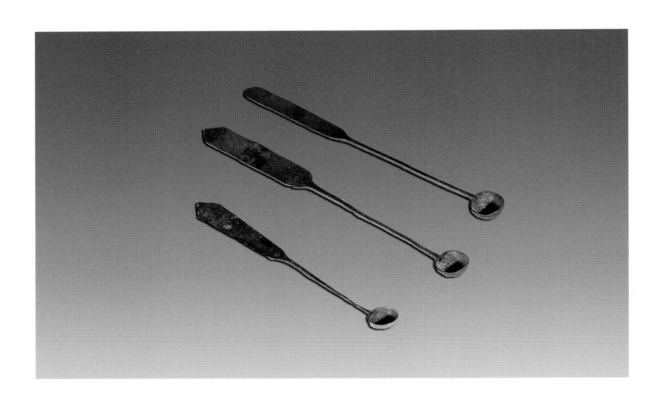

蒙医药勺

清

铜质

柄长分别为 16.5 厘米、23 厘米、23.5 厘米

勺径分别为 1.8 厘米、2.2 厘米、2.4 厘米

Mongolian Medicine Spoons

Qing Dynasty

Copper

Handle Length 16.5 cm, 23 cm, and 23.5 cm respectively

Spoon Diameter 1.8 cm, 2.2cm, and 2.4 cm respectively

蒙医量药用具，从蒙药袋内取量药粉之用。半球形勺，细长颈，斜肩，扁平柄，柄端上者为弧形，中、下者为尖形。

中国医史博物馆藏

These spoons were used by Mongolian doctors to take out and measure medicinal powders from the medicine bags. The spoon heads are half rounded, and the slim necks slope into flat handles with triangular ends.

Preserved in Chinese Medical History Museum

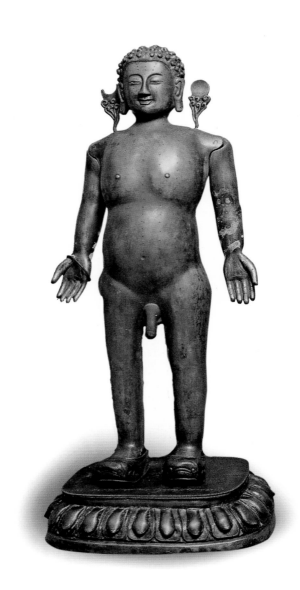

蒙医针灸铜人

晚清

铜质

身高 61 厘米

蒙医针灸铜人原系已故北京雍和宫喇嘛邰元真收藏之物，1957 年赠予内蒙古呼和浩特市中蒙医研究所。制作年代不详，铜人底座上刻有藏文"十六□□庚辰年造"。此件为复制品，原件双肩上的日月佚失。

北京中医药大学中医药博物馆藏

Mongolian Copper Acupuncture Figurine

Late Qing Dynasty

Copper

Height 61 cm

The figurine was collected by Tai Yuanzhen, a late lama of Yonghegong Lamasery in Beijing, who donated it to the Chinese and Mongolian Medicine Research Institute, Hohhot, Inner Mongolia Autonomous Region in 1957. It is still unknown when it was made, though its Bottom is carved with "Made in 16 □□ " in Mongolian. This piece is a replica. The moon and the sun on the original's shoulders were missing.

Preserved in The Museum of Chinese Medicine, Beijing University of Chinese Medicine

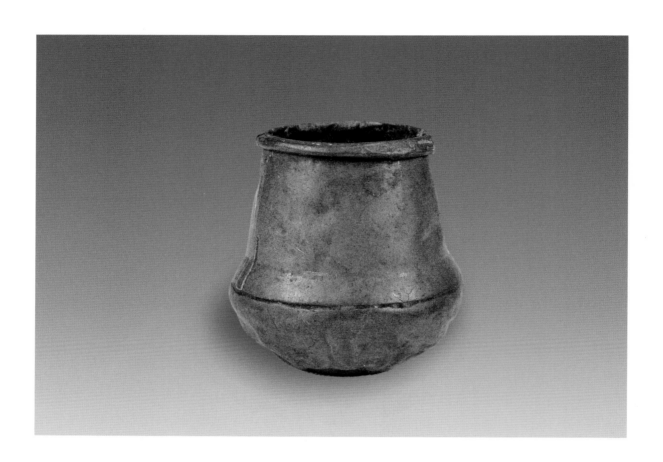

紫铜拔火罐

清

紫铜质

底径 3.4 厘米，高 5 厘米

Red Copper Cupping Cup

Qing Dynasty

Red Copper

Bottom Diameter 3.4 cm/ Height 5 cm

藏医、蒙医传统的拔火罐。1978 年在内蒙古
包头采集。

陕西医史博物馆藏

The cup was utilized for cupping therapy by
traditional Tibetan and Mongolian doctors.
It was collected in Baotou, Inner Mongolia
Autonomous Region in 1978.
Preserved in Shaanxi Museum of Medical History

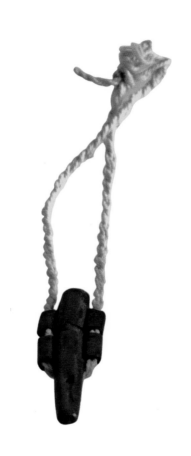

铜针筒

清

铜质

长 7 厘米，直径 1.2 厘米

Copper Needle Holder

Qing Dynasty

Copper

Length 7 cm/ Diameter 1.2 cm

仫佬族用具。罗城东门镇佑洞村征集。

罗城仫佬族博物馆藏

The needle was used by the Mulao. It was collected at Youdong Village, Dongmen Town, Luocheng Mulao Autonomous County, Guangxi Zhuang Autonomous Region.

Preserved in Luocheng Mulao Museum

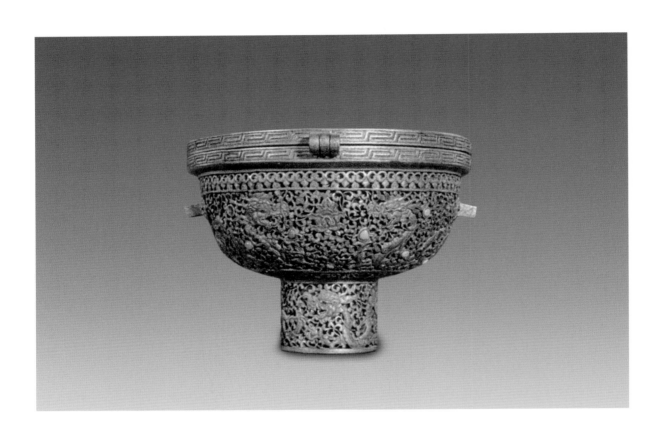

镶绿松石镀金铜质龙纹高足碗套

19 世纪

铜质

口径 18 厘米，底径 6.2 厘米，高 13 厘米

Gilded Copper Stem Bowl Wrapper Inlaid with Calaite and Decorated with Dragon Patterns

19th Century

Copper

Mouth Diameter 18 cm/ Bottom Diameter 6.2 cm/ Height 13 cm

通体鎏金，遍饰装饰图案，套身上透雕双龙
戏珠和花草纹纹饰，底部錾有双龙戏珠，局
部镶有精美的绿松石。碗套具有保护瓷器，
降低瓷器在运输过程中破损率的作用。具有
浓厚的民族文化特征。

西藏博物馆藏

Thoroughly gilded in gold and fully decorated,
the wrapper is inlaid with two dragons playing
with a pearl and patterns of flora on the body.
On the Bottom are also engraved two dragons
playing with a pearl. It is partially inlaid with
calaite. The wrapper was used to protect the
porcelain bowl in transportation. The ethnic
culture features prominently on the bowl
wrapper.

Preserved in Tibet Museum

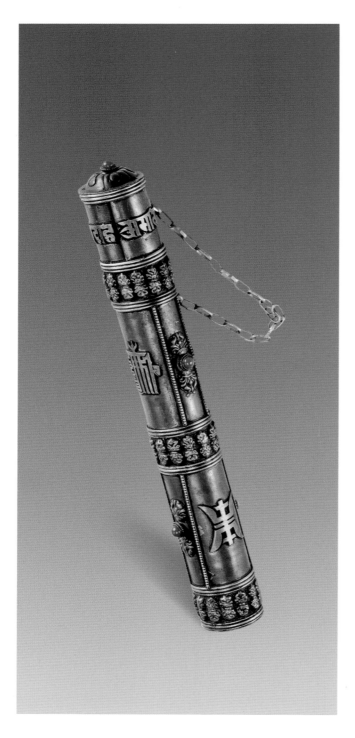

经书筒

近现代

铜质

长 28 厘米

用于珍藏医疗经典。

内蒙古国际蒙医蒙药博物馆藏

Scripture Holder

Modern Times

Copper

Length 28 cm

It was used to conserve medical classics.

Preserved in Inner Mongolia International

Mongolian Medicine Museum

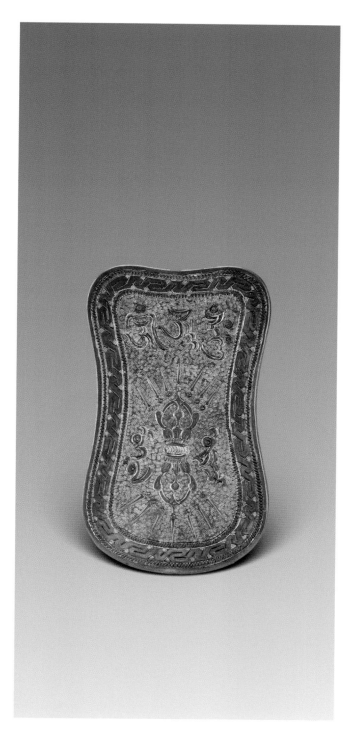

蒙藏文铜按摩器

现代

铜质

长 12 厘米

用于按摩治疗。

内蒙古医科大学蒙医药博物馆藏

Copper Massager with Mongolian and Tibetan Inscriptions

Modern Times

Copper

Length 12 cm

It was used in massage therapy.

Preserved in the Mongolian Medicine Museum

of Inner Mongolia Medical University

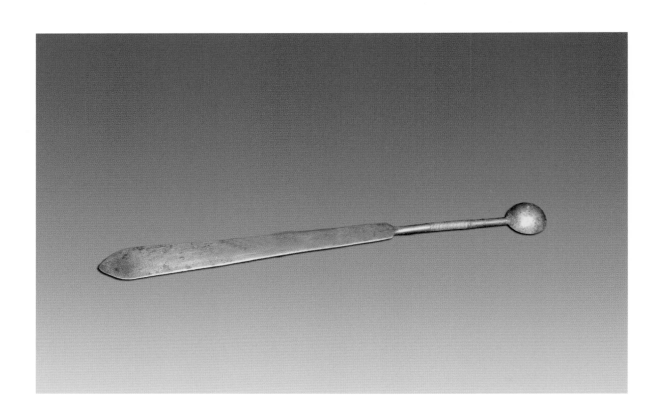

蒙医药勺

近代

铜质

长 21.5 厘米，勺径 2 厘米，重 25 克

Mongolian Medicine Spoon

Modern Times

Copper

Length 21.5 cm/ Spoon Diameter 2 cm/ Weight 25 g

勺头小深，接勺头处细圆，后柄呈扁平状。

医药器具。完整无损。

陕西医史博物馆藏

The spoon is small but deep with a slim rod connected to a flat handle. It was for medical use, and is still in good condition.

Preserved in Shaanxi Museum of Medical History

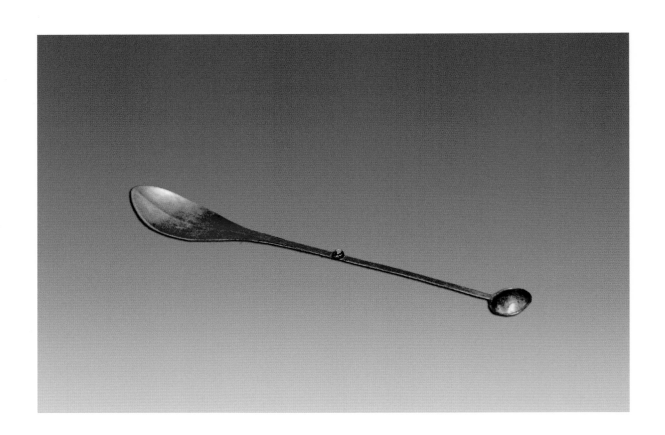

铜药勺

铜质

长 21 厘米

Copper Medicine Spoon

Copper

Length 21 cm

传世品。药勺一端为圆勺，另一端为树叶状
扁平勺，可秤取不同剂量的药物。勺柄的中
间还镶有一孔雀石。药勺既是取药工具，又
是量具。西藏拉萨征集。

北京中医药大学中医药博物馆藏

The spoon is handed down from ancient times.
It is double-headed, with a round head at one
end and a flat leaf-shaped head at the other. The
center of the handle is inlaid with a grain of
malachite. This medicine spoon was a tool for
taking out and measuring medicinal powders.
It was collected in Lhasa, Tibet Autonomous
Region.

Preserved in The Museum of Chinese Medicine,
Beijing University of Chinese Medicine

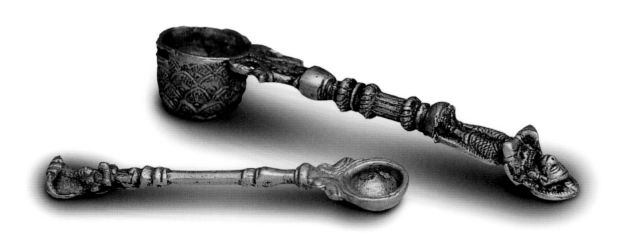

月王铜药勺

铜质

大者长 20.5 厘米，勺口径 3.5 厘米，勺深 3.5 厘米

小者长 15 厘米，勺口径 2.2 厘米，勺深 1.5 厘米

Copper Medicine Spoons with Sculptures of Moon King

Copper

The bigger one: Length 20.5 cm/ Spoon Diameter 3.5 cm/ Spoon Depth 3.5 cm

The smaller one: Length 15 cm/ Spoon Diameter 2.2 cm/ Spoon Depth 1.5 cm

传世品。大勺的外部刻有荷花瓣花纹，勺柄另一端铸有藏族崇敬的古代月王像；小勺把的另一端月王像头上铸有一弯曲的手掌形药勺，两端可分别取用不同剂量的药末。藏医取药用具。甘肃省甘南藏族自治州征集。

北京中医药大学中医药博物馆藏

These spoons are handed down from ancient times. The bigger one is decorated with lotus petals on the outside and cast with a sculpture of the popularly-worshiped ancient Moon King at the end of the handle. On the head of the smaller Moon King is a medicinal ladle in the shape of a curved palm. Both ends of the smaller spoon were utilized for taking out and measuring medicinal powders. As Tibetan medicine tools, they were collected in Gannan Tibetan Autonomous Prefecture, Gansu Province.

Preserved in The Museum of Chinese Medicine, Beijing University of Chinese Medicine

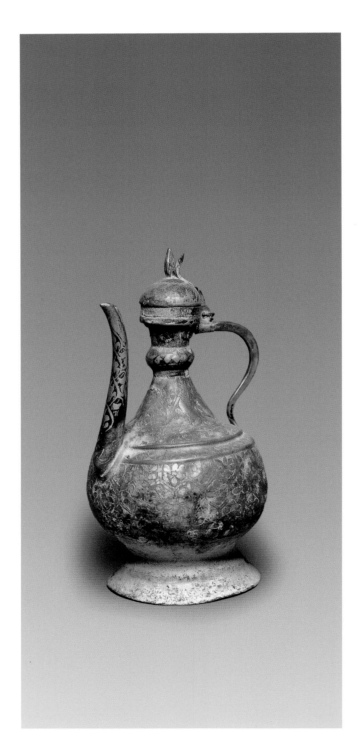

洗手壶

铜质

口径 5 厘米，腹径 16 厘米，高 30.5 厘米

Hand-washing Pot

Copper

Mouth Diameter 5 cm/ Belly Diameter 16 cm/

Height 30.5 cm

锥形长颈，扁鼓腹，高圈足，壶嘴细长高于壶口，壶盖上有一四棱尖锥形錾，壶身上刻有传统的阿拉伯花纹，壶手柄上端用阿拉伯文刻有"1350"字样。维吾尔族洗手用具。新疆喀什征集。

北京中医药大学中医药博物馆藏

The pot has a cone-shaped bottleneck, a flat bulging body and a high foot ring with its thin spout higher than its mouth. There is a rectangular pyramid-shaped handle on its lid. On its body are carved traditional arabesque, and on its body handle are the carved Arabic numerals "1350". The pot was utilized for hand washing by the Uygur people. It was collected in Kashi, Xinjiang Uygur Autonomous Region. Preserved in The Museum of Chinese Medicine, Beijing University of Chinese Medicine

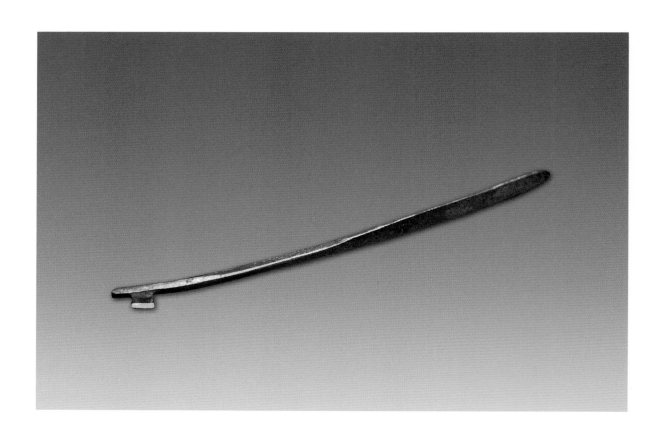

放血刀

铜质

长 11 厘米

Fleam

Copper

Length 11 cm

传世品。藏医和蒙医"放血疗法"的主要用具。
内蒙古阿拉善左旗征集。

北京中医药大学中医药博物馆藏

This fleam is handed down from ancient times.
It was a major instrument for blood-letting
therapy by the Tibetan and Mongolian doctors.
It was collected in Alxa Left Banner, Inner
Mongolia Autonomous Region.
Preserved in The Museum of Chinese Medicine,
Beijing University of Chinese Medicine

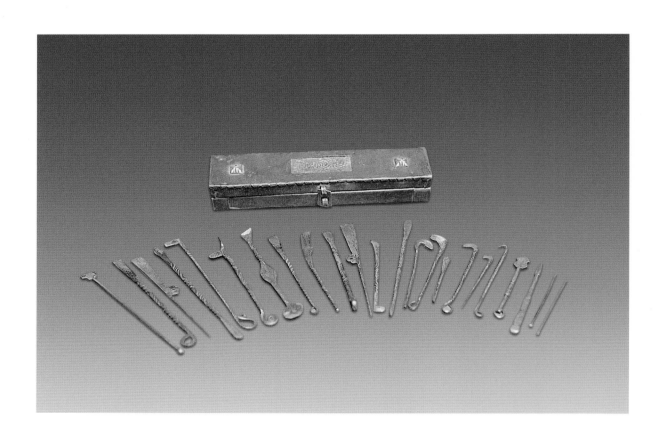

医疗器具

铜质

最长 15.5 厘米，最短 9 厘米

Medical Instruments

Copper

Maximum Length 15.5 cm/ Minimum Length 9 cm

23件。传世品。藏医医疗手术用具，包括刀、钩、针、匙等。上为用具箱。甘肃省甘南藏族自治州征集。

北京中医药大学中医药博物馆藏

These 23 pieces are handed down from ancient times, including knives, hamuli, needles, scoops, etc. On the upper part of this picture is the toolkit. They were collected in Gannan Tibetan Autonomous Prefecture, Gansu Province.

Preserved in The Museum of Chinese Medicine, Beijing University of Chinese Medicine

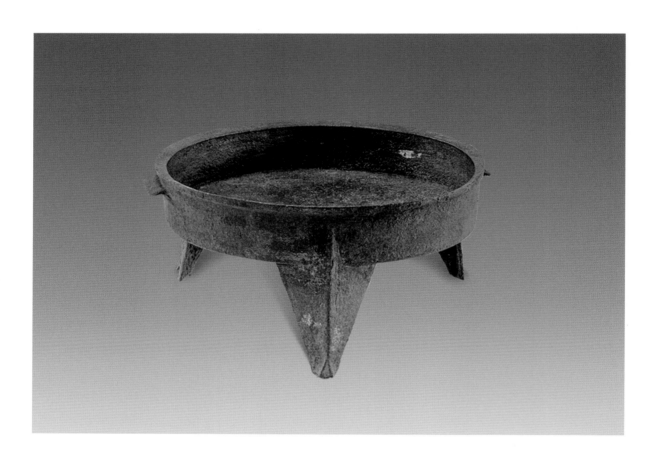

三足双耳铁撑

元

铁质

口径 41.5 厘米，通宽 45.5 厘米，高 21 厘米

Three-legged Double-handled Iron Pot

Yuan Dynasty

Iron

Mouth Diameter 41.5 cm/ Width 45.5 cm/ Height 21 cm

铸造。侈口，双耳，浅直腹，平底，三锥形高足。
蒙古族烹调面食用的炊具。内蒙古乌兰察布
市察右前旗出土。

内蒙古博物院藏

This iron casting is wide-mouthed and double-
handled with a shallow and straight belly, a
flat bottom, and three long tampering legs.
Mongolians used it to cook flour food. It was
excavated at Chayouqian Banner, Wulanchabu
City, Inner Mongolia Autonomous Region.
Preserved in Inner Mongolia Museum

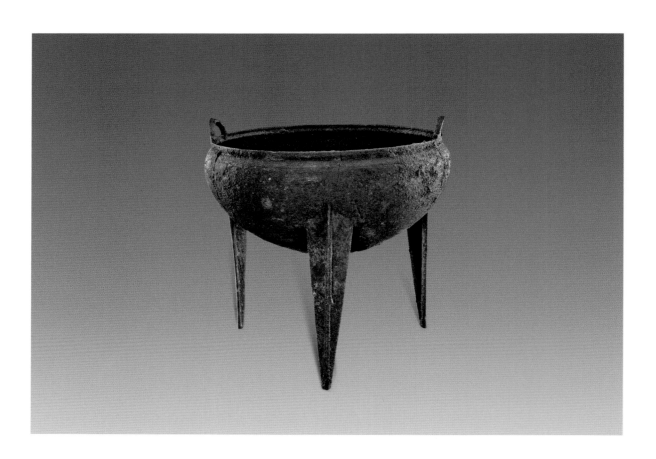

三尖足铁锅

元

铁质

高 47 厘米

Three-legged Iron Pot

Yuan Dynasty

Iron

Height 47 cm

铸造。敞口，双环耳，深鼓腹，尖底，三锥
形高足。蒙古族烹调肉食用的炊具。内蒙古
乌兰察布市察右前旗出土。

内蒙古博物院藏

This iron casting is wide-mouthed with two ring
handles, a deep bulging belly, a cone bottom,
and three long tampering legs. Mongolians
used it to cook meat food. It was excavated at
Chayouqian Banner, Wulanchabu City, Inner
Mongolia Autonomous Region.

Preserved in Inner Mongolia Museum

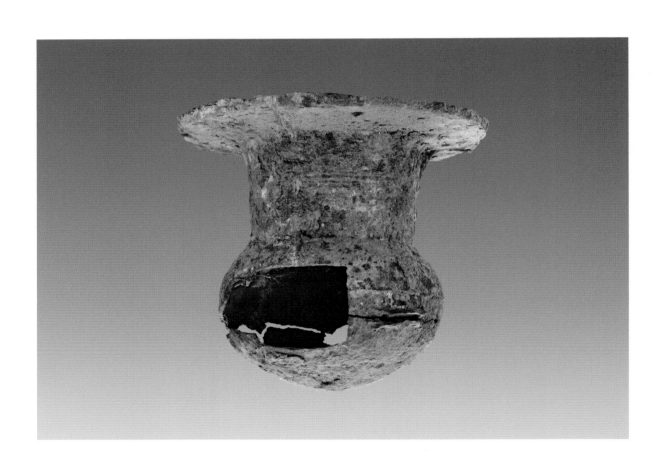

铁煤炉

元

铁质

盘宽 47.5 厘米，高 59 厘米

Iron Stove

Yuan Dynasty

Iron

Width 47.5 cm/ Height 59 cm

烧煤的炉子。平折沿宽而厚，上部为圆柱形，下部圆鼓，有长方形炉口，三圈足（已经朽坏）。北京市海淀区西直门后英房胡同出土。出土时，在炉盘上垫支五块碎砖头，由于火烤的缘故，砖头已经变为土红色。

首都博物馆藏

It was used to burn coals. It has a wide and thick flat folding edge, a cylindrical upper part, a drum-shaped lower part, a rectangular mouth and three ring feet (already rotten). It was unearthed in Houyingfang Hutong, Xizhimen Street, Haidian District, Beijing City. When it was unearthed, five broken bricks supporting the stove plate had become soil red due to the fire.

Preserved in The Capital Museum

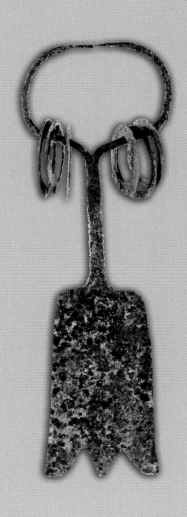

三叉状萨满法器

元

铁质

通长 60 厘米，宽 18 厘米

长铲形，前端三齿，柄首为如意云纹圈，上穿六个铁环，是萨满做法时手持的法器。

内蒙古博物院藏

Trident Shaman Magic Instrument

Yuan Dynasty

Iron

Length 60 cm/ Width 18 cm

The long-shovel-shaped instrument has three teeth at its head and six iron rings with patterns of Ruyi moire rings at the end of the handle. It was used by Shamans for their practicing.

Preserved in Inner Mongolia Museum

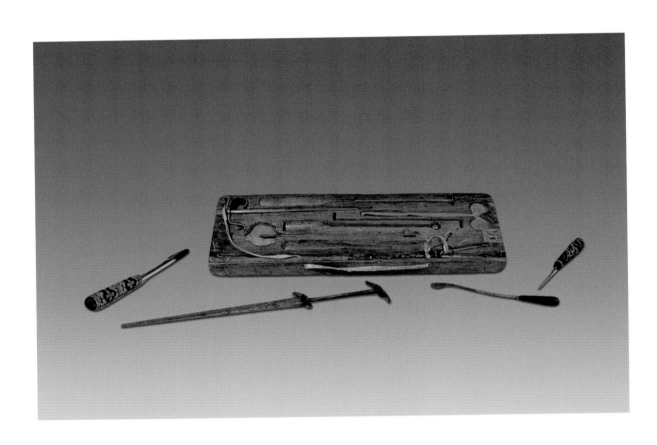

铁制医疗器械

17 世纪

铁质

Iron Medical Instruments

17th Century

Iron

11件套，包括穿刺针、刀、剪子、镊子等器械，做工精良，有的执柄上绘有精美的纹饰，配有精美的木盒。

西藏博物馆藏

There are 11 pieces in this set of medical instruments, including puncture needles, scalpels, scissors, tweezers, etc. All the delicate pieces, some of which are decorated with exquisite patterns on the handle, are stored in a fine wooden case.

Preserved in Tibet Museum

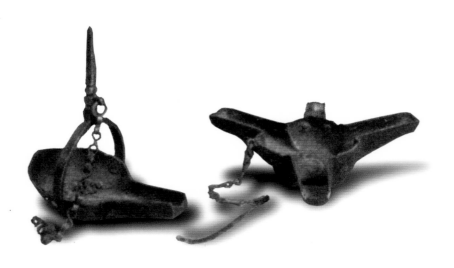

铁质莲瓣形油灯和船形油灯

19 世纪

铁质

莲瓣形宽 25 厘米，高 5.8 厘米

船形宽 16.5 厘米，高 18.4 厘米

西藏博物馆藏

Lotus Petal-shaped and Boat-shaped Iron Oil Lamps

19th Century

Iron

Lotus petal-shaped iron oil lamp: Width 25 cm/ Height 5.8 cm

Boat-shaped iron oil lamp: Width 16.5 cm/ Height 18.4 cm

Preserved in Tibet Museum

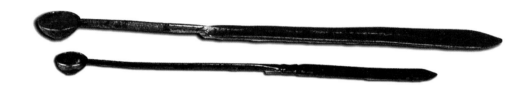

蒙医药勺

清

铁质

大者长 16.5 厘米，勺径 1.5 厘米

小者长 12.6 厘米，勺径 1.4 厘米

蒙医量药用具，一端为半球形勺，扁长柄，柄端为钝角形。1978 年内蒙古包头五当召洛勃桑活佛赠。

陕西医史博物馆藏

Mongolian Medicine Spoons

Qing Dynasty

Iron

The bigger one: Length 16.5 cm/ Spoon Diameter 1.5 cm

The smaller one: Length 12.6 cm/ Spoon Diameter 1.4 cm

The spoons were used by Mongolian doctors to take out and measure medicinal powders. The spoon heads are half round, held by flat blunt-ended handles. They were presented by a living Buddha from Baotou, Inner Mongolia Autonomous Region in 1978.

Preserved in Shaanxi Museum of Medical History

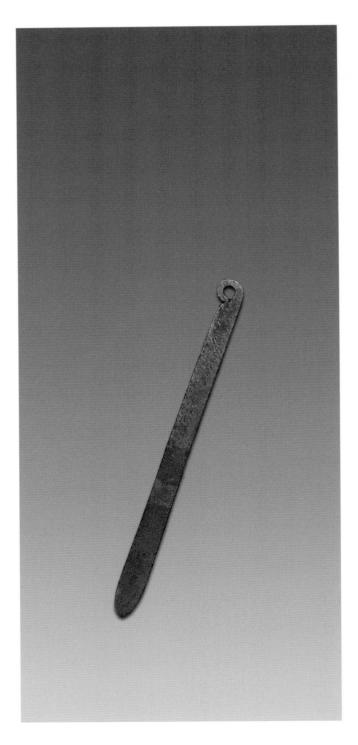

切开排脓工具

清

铁质

通长 7.7 厘米，宽 0.6 厘米，厚 0.15 厘米

Instrument for the Incision and Drainage of Pustules

Qing Dynasty

Iron

Length 7.7 cm/ Width 0.6 cm/ Thickness 0.15 cm

长扁形，一端有系孔，用作切开脓疱、排引脓流的工具，为外科手术用具。保存基本完好。此为通过自购收藏的清末少数民族外科手术工具之一。

中华医学会/上海中医药大学医史博物馆藏

This long and flat surgical knife was utilized for the incision and drainage of pustules. It has a tie hole at one end. Collected by means of buying, this late Qing Dynasty minority surgical instrument is still in good condition.

Preserved in Chinese Medical Association/ Museum of Chinese Medicine, Shanghai University of Traditional Chinese Medicine

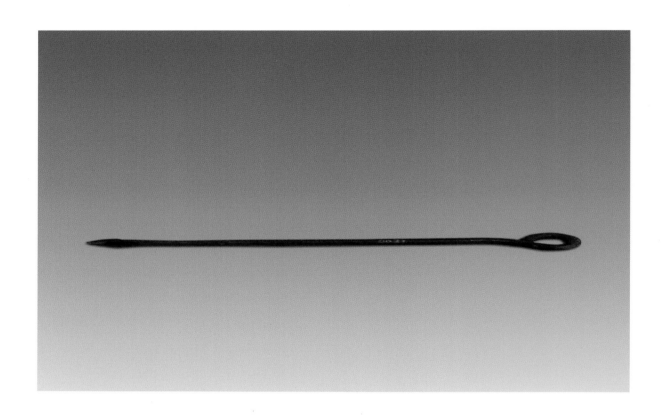

彝族痈刀

近代

铁质

长 21 厘米，重 150 克

Yi's Scalpel for Carbuncle Draining

Modern Times

Iron

Length 21 cm/ Weight 150 g

尖为菱形，手把为圆形。制药（治疗）工具。

完整无损。四川省凉山彝族自治州征集。

陕西医史博物馆藏

Sharp-ended with a rod handle, the knife was
used for medical purpose. It is still in good
condition. It was collected in Liangshan Yi
Autonomous Prefecture, Sichuan Province.
Preserved in Shaanxi Museum of Medical History

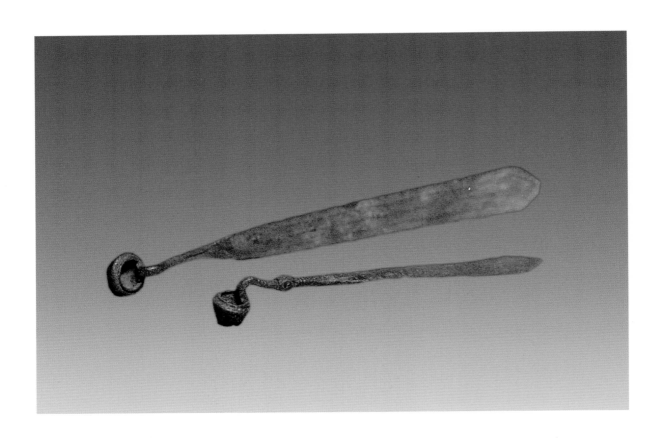

蒙医药勺

铁质

分别长 30 厘米、23 厘米

Mongolian Medicine Spoons

Iron

Length 30 cm and 23 cm respectively

传世品。勺头呈半圆形，勺柄前窄后宽，勺
与柄间以弧形相连。蒙医取药粉的用具。内
蒙古阿拉善左旗征集。

北京中医药大学中医药博物馆藏

The spoon heads are half rounded. Holding
the head by curved necks, the handles extend
increasingly wider to the other end. The spoons
are handed down from ancient Mongolian
doctors who used them to take out and measure
medicine powders. They were collected in
Alxa Left Banner, Inner Mongolia Autonomous
Region.

Preserved in The Museum of Chinese Medicine,
Beijing University of Chinese Medicine

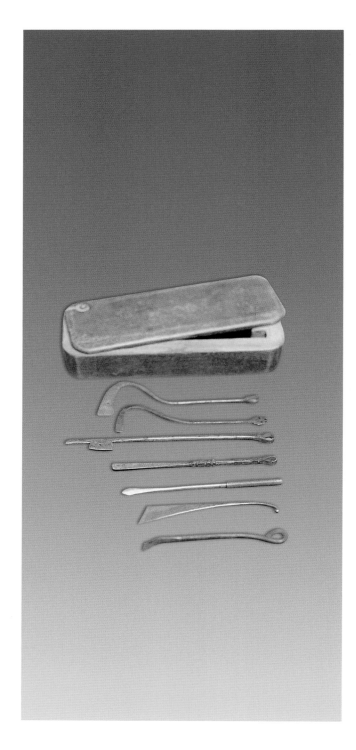

藏医手术器具

金属质

最长 15.5 厘米，最短 9 厘米

Tibetan Surgical Instruments

Metal

Maximum Length 15.5 cm/ Minimum Length 9 cm

7件。从上至下为1~7号，其中5号为穿刺针，余为各种手术刀。甘肃省甘南藏族自治州征集。

北京中医药大学中医药博物馆藏

These seven pieces are numbered from 1 to 7 from top to bottom. No. 5 is a puncture needle, while the others are scalpels. They were collected in Gannan Tibetan Autonomous Prefecture, Gansu Province.
Preserved in The Museum of Chinese Medicine, Beijing University of Chinese Medicine

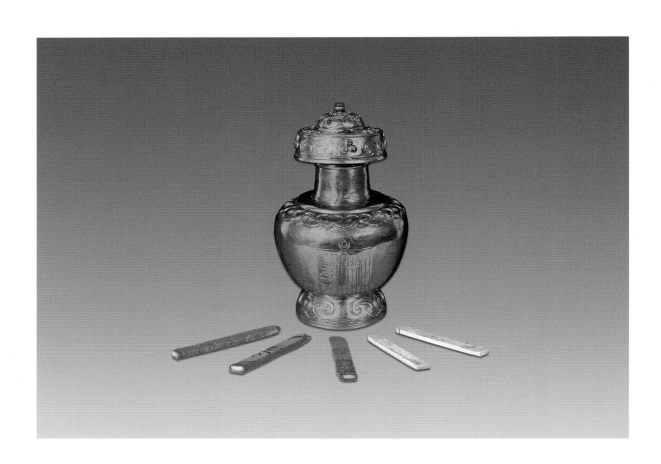

金本巴瓶

清·乾隆

金质

最大直径 22.7 厘米，底径 14.5 厘米，高 34 厘米

Gold Bumba Bottle

Qianlong Period, Qing Dynasty

Gold

Maximum Diameter 22.7 cm/ Bottom Diameter 14.5 cm/ Height 34 cm

铸造。铸以莲瓣如意头、缠枝等纹饰，盖上镶红珊瑚和蓝宝石，瓶口内插签筒，签筒内放置如意头象牙签 5 支。

西藏博物馆藏

The bottle is cast with ornaments of Ruyi lotus petals and interlaced flora. The cover is inlaid with red coral and sapphires. The bottle mouth is filled with a lot pot, in which five Ruyi ivory lots are laid.

Preserved in Tibet Museum

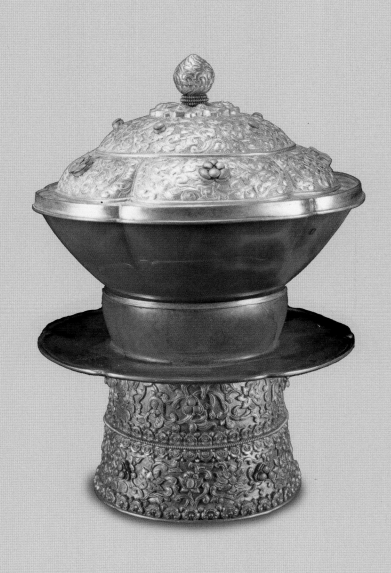

金嵌玛瑙碗

清

金质

高 19.3 厘米

全器采用錾刻、镶嵌技术，工艺精湛，兼具满、蒙、藏三种风格。碗刻"寿"字，足刻乾隆款。

故宫博物院藏

Agate-inlaid Gold Bowl

Qing Dynasty

Gold

Height 19.3 cm

The bowl is prettily engraved and inlaid. It is a perfect combination of Manchu, Tibetan and Mongolian styles. On the bowl is carved a the Chinese character "Shou" (longevity), and on the foot is the inscription "Qianlong".

Preserved in The Palace Museum

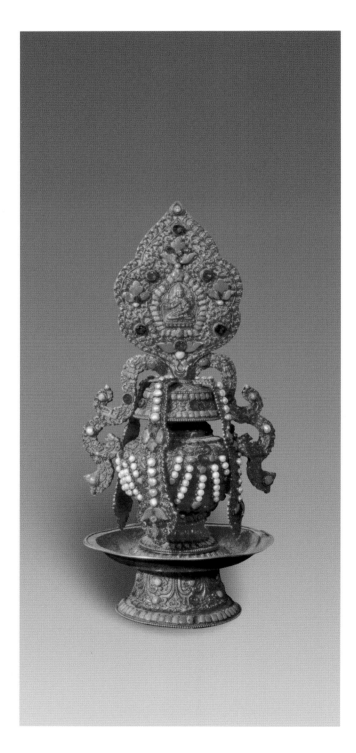

镶宝石金质长寿瓶

19 世纪

金质

宽 14.8 厘米，底径 8.8 厘米，高 29.3 厘米

Gemmed Gold Bottle of Longevity

19th Century

Gold

Width 14.8 cm/ Bottom Diameter 8.8 cm/

Height 29.3 cm

由托盘、瓶身和瓶盖三部分组成。瓶盖样式
复杂，錾刻无量寿佛。长寿瓶各部分均饰有
莲瓣和卷草纹，并镶嵌珍珠、绿松石和红宝
石，是藏传佛教举行隆重的灌顶仪式时必备
的法器之一。

西藏博物馆藏

This set consists of a tray, a bottle, and a
cover. On the intricately-designed cover sits an
engraved Buddha of Longevity in meditation.
The bottle is fully decorated with patterns of
lotus petals and floral scrolls, and gemmed
with pearls, johnites, and rubies. It is an
indispensable ritual instrument at Abhisheka of
Tibetan Buddhism.

Preserved in Tibet Museum

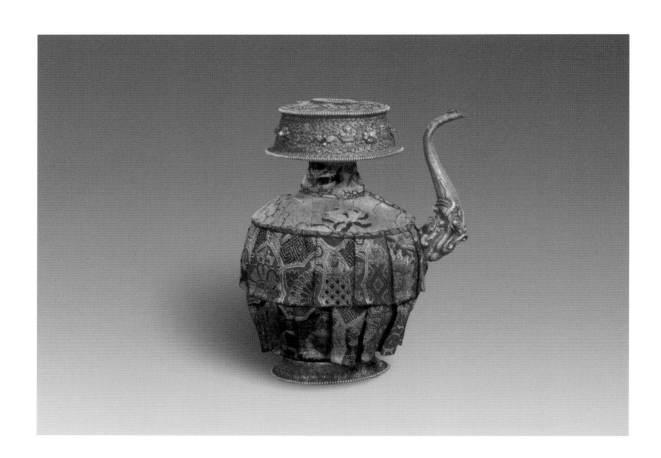

镶宝石金质净水瓶

19 世纪

金质

口径 8.8 厘米，宽 19.3 厘米，底径 4.4 厘米，高 22.5 厘米

Gemmed Gold Water Bottle

19th Century

Gold

Mouth Diameter 8.8 cm/ Width 19.3 cm/ Bottom Diameter 4.4 cm/ Height 22.5 cm

束颈，溜肩，鼓腹，圈足微外撇，前有龙首形流，盖上饰八宝和瑞草纹，镶嵌珊瑚和绿松石。用于盛神水——用清水泡以藏红花，洒圣水盛给信徒倒少许，作为加持水。此瓶是举行宗教活动时为神像或信徒进行沐浴时所用的器物。

西藏博物馆藏

The bottle is featured with a convergent neck, sloping shoulders, a bulging body, a slightly outstretching foot, and a dragon-shaped spout. The cover is decorated with patterns of Eight Treasures and auspicious herbs, and gemmed with coral and johnites. As a vessel for the holy water – the blessed fresh water soaked with dried crocuses which will be sprayed or poured a little bit on the heads of the Buddha's followers, it is a ritual instrument for the bathing of Buddha statues or the followers.
Preserved in Tibet Museum

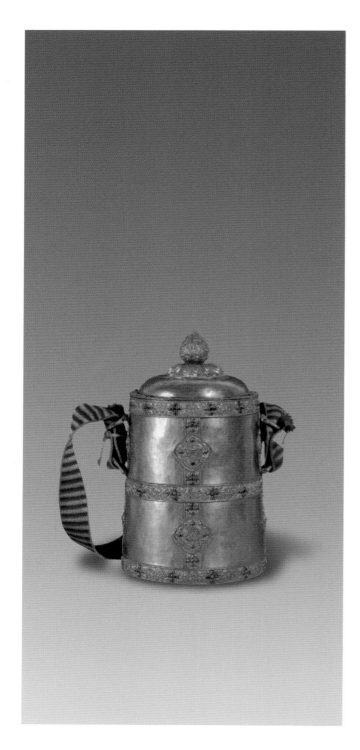

镶绿松石金质盛食桶

20 世纪初

金质

口径 18 厘米，底径 25 厘米，高 35 厘米

Turquoise-inlaid Gold Food Bucket

Early 20th Century

Gold

Mouth Diameter 18 cm/ Bottom Diameter 25 cm/

Height 35 cm

圆柱形，子母口，带盖，宝塔钮，对耳，耳上系带，平底，圈足，镶绿松石，盛食用。贵族生活用品。

西藏博物馆藏

The cylinder-shaped bucket has a synthesized set of mouths, a flat bottom, a ring foot, a lid, a pagoda-shaped knob and two ears on which a strap is tied. As a daily life article used by the nobility to keep food, it is inlaid with calaite.

Preserved in Tibet Museum

镶宝石金质沐浴壶

20 世纪初

金质镶宝石

宽 10 厘米，高 20 厘米

沐浴壶，又称"奔巴壶"，系藏传佛教仪式
盛净水用。这种壶的造型一般分为壶盖、壶
腹、壶座、壶嘴，覆钵式壶盖和壶座，壶座
略内收，精细致极。

西藏博物馆藏

Gemmed Gold Bath Pot

Early 20th Century

Gemmed Gold

Width 10 cm/ Height 20 cm

The bath pot, also named "Bumba pot", is used
to hold holy water at Tibetan Buddhism rituals.
Such pots generally have a cover, a spout, a
body and a foot. With an overlapping cover and
a convergent foot, the pot is quite exquisite.

Preserved in Tibet Museum

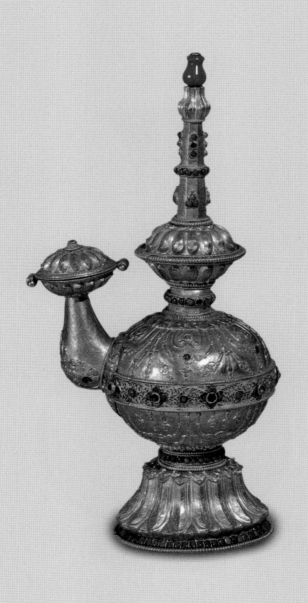

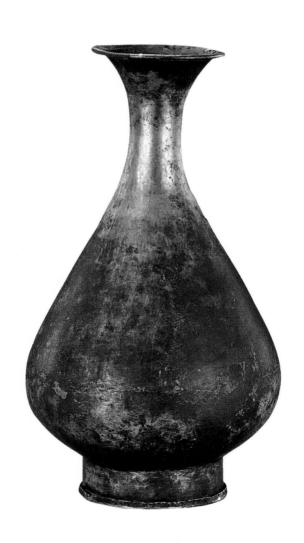

银玉壶春瓶

元

银质

口径 7.8 厘米，底径 8.8 厘米，高 27.5 厘米

喇叭口，细颈，垂腹，圈足。元代蒙古族典型酒具。内蒙古鄂尔多斯市征集。

内蒙古博物院藏

Silver Yuhuchun-style Bottle

Yuan Dynasty

Silver

Mouth Diameter 7.8 cm/ Bottom Diameter 8.8 cm/
Height 27.5 cm

With a trumpet-shaped mouth, a slim neck, a drooping belly and a round foot, this bottle was a Mongolian drinking vessel in the Yuan Dynasty. It was collected in Ordos City, Inner Mongolia Autonomous Region.

Preserved in Inner Mongolia Museum

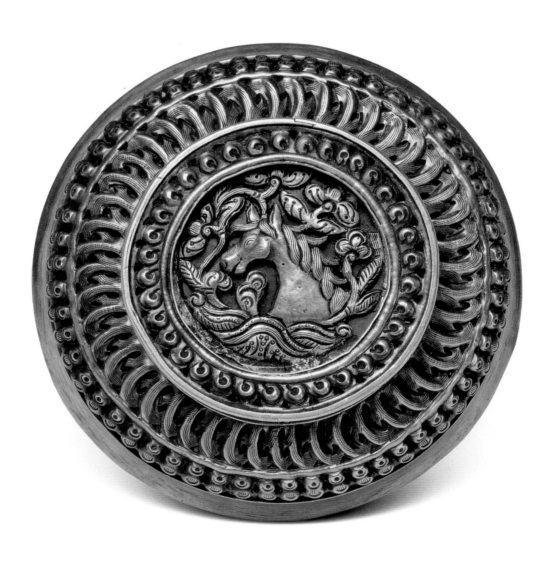

银碗

清

银质

口径 12.5 厘米

用于饮食疗法。

内蒙古博物院藏

Silver Bowl

Qing Dynasty

Silver

Mouth Diameter 12.5 cm

It was used in diet therapy.

Preserved in Inner Mongolia Museum

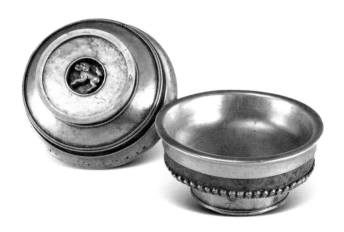

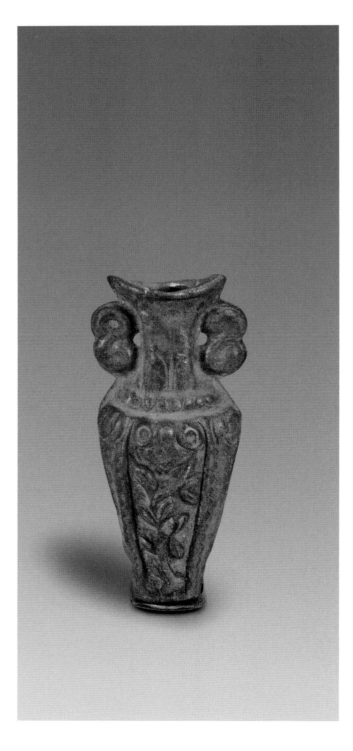

蒙医银药瓶

清

银质

高 6 厘米

Mongolian Silver Medicine Bottle

Qing Dynasty

Silver

Height 6 cm

弧形口，口沿厚而微外撇，束颈，带"乙"型
对耳，溜肩，腹微收至足，平底，圈足，器
身上刻有花纹。盛药器具。在内蒙古包头市
采集。

陕西医史博物馆藏

The arc-shaped mouth is thickly brimmed
and slightly outstretched. The neck is set with
two inverted-S-shaped handles. From the
sloping shoulder, the belly contracts gently to
the flat rounded foot. The top of the bottle is
carved with patterns. It was used as a medicine
container. It was collected in Baotou, Inner
Mongolia Autonomous Region.

Preserved in Shaanxi Museum of Medical History

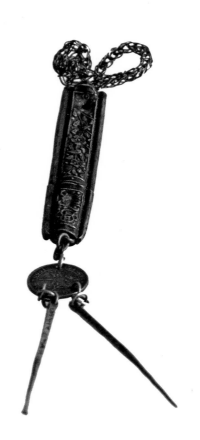

银针筒

清

银质

长 20 厘米，直径 1.5 厘米

Silver Needle Holder

Qing Dynasty

Silver

Length 20 cm/ Diameter 1.5 cm

仫佬族用具。罗城东门镇佑洞村征集。

罗城仫佬族博物馆藏

The holder was used by the Mulao. It was collected at Youdong Village, Dongmen Town, Luocheng Mulao Autonomous County, Guangxi Zhuang Autonomous Region.

Preserved in Luocheng Mulao Museum

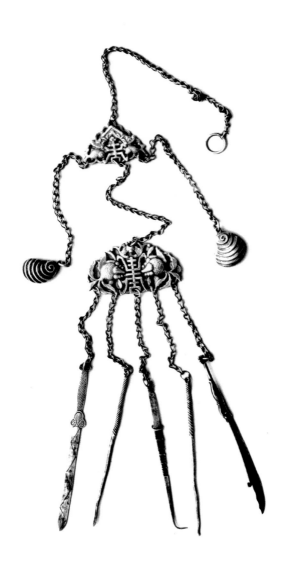

"福寿"型银五配件

清

银质

总长 68 厘米，最宽处 8 厘米

仫佬族佩饰，既能驱邪，又是卫生方面的实
用品。罗城东门镇东西街传世品。

陈昌炽藏

Silver Accessories of Happiness and Longevity (Five Pieces)

Qing Dynasty

Silver

Length 68 cm/ Maximum Width 8 cm

The Mulao wore the accessories to expel evil
spirits and keep health. It is a precious heritage
of Dongxi Street, Dongmen Town, Luocheng
Mulao Autonomous County.

Collected by Chen Changchi

蝴蝶型银驱邪挂件

清

银质

长 39 厘米，宽 9.8 厘米

仫佬族佩饰，用于驱邪。罗城东门镇横岸村
征集。

罗城仫佬族博物馆藏

Butterfly-shaped Exorcism Silver Accessory

Qing Dynasty

Silver

Length 39 cm/ Width 9.8 cm

The Mulao wore the accessory to expel evil
spirits. It was collected at Heng'an Village in
Dongmen Town, Luocheng Mulao Autonomous
County.

Preserved in Luocheng Mulao Museum

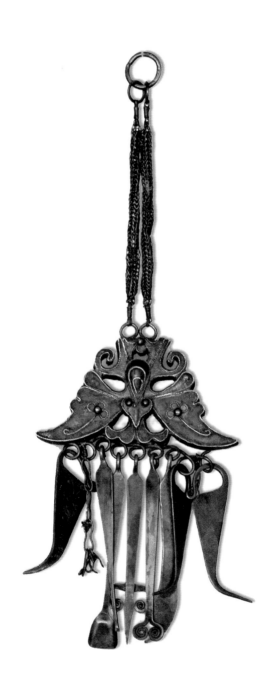

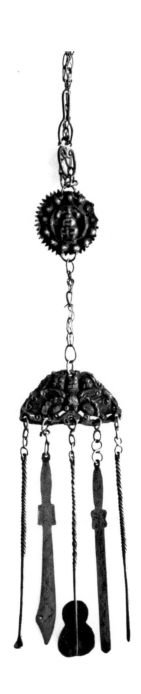

蝴蝶型银五配件

清

银质

总长 28 厘米，最宽处 6.5 厘米

仫佬族佩饰，既能驱邪，又是卫生方面的实用品。罗城乔善乡古金村征集。

陈昌炽藏

Butterfly-shaped Exorcism Silver Accessories (Five Pieces)

Qing Dynasty

Silver

Length 28 cm/ Maximum Width 6.5 cm

The Mulao wore the accessories to expel evil spirits and keep health. It was collected at Gujin Village, Qiaoshan Town, Luocheng Mulao Autonomous County.

Collected by Chen Changchi

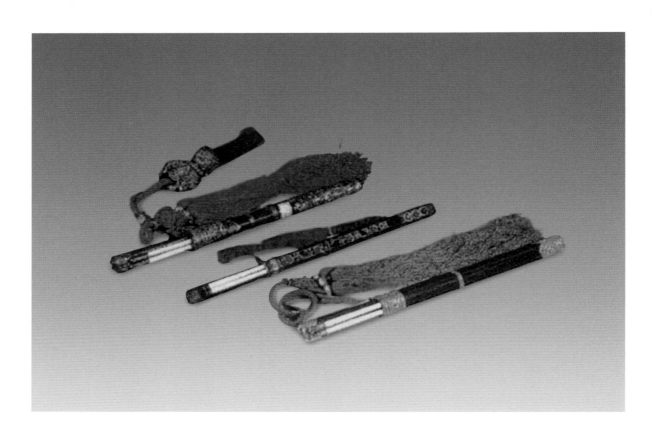

蒙古刀、筷

19 世纪

最长 33.5 厘米

Mongolian Knives and Chopsticks

19th Century

Maximum Length 33.5 cm

蒙古刀、筷是蒙古族的生活用具，经常戴在身上，既是牧民不可缺少的日用品，又是一种装饰品。在蒙古人心中，蒙古刀是腾格里所赐的圣物，象征着给自己和身边朋友带来好运和平安。随身携带的蒙古筷子是蒙古人民注重饮食卫生的标志。

西藏博物馆藏

Mongolians usually carry knives and chopsticks for daily use, which are indispensable for their life and ornamental purposes. To Mongolians, knives are holy gifts bestowed by Tengger as symbols of fortune and safety. The carry-on chopsticks indicate that Mongolians are strict with food hygiene.

Preserved in Tibet Museum

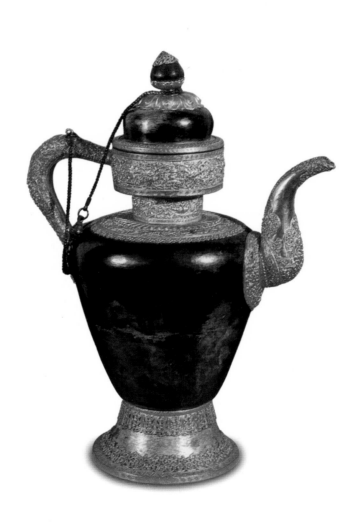

包金银净水壶

20 世纪初

银质包金

宽 60 厘米，高 68 厘米

有提，短流，盖和提之间有连接，器型优美。

盛水器具。

西藏博物馆藏

Gilded Silver Water Pot

Early 20th Century

Gilded Silver

Width 60 cm/ Height 68 cm

The elegantly-shaped water pot has a short
spout, and a handle tied to the cover.

Preserved in Tibet Museum

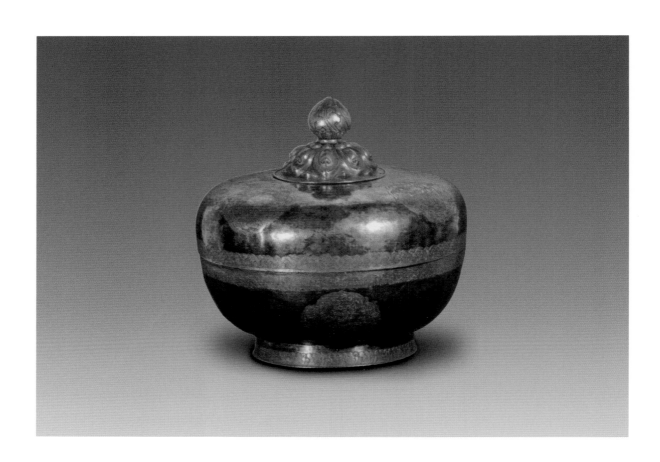

鎏金錾花银质盛食盖盒

20 世纪

银质

口径 34 厘米，底径 21.5 厘米，高 33 厘米

Flower-inlaid Gilded Silver Hamper

20th Century

Silver

Mouth Diameter 34 cm/ Bottom Diameter 21.5 cm/ Height 33 cm

扁圆形，子母口，带钮，平底，圈足，磨光，鎏金錾花。贵族生活用品。

西藏博物馆藏

The oblate hamper has a snap-lid, a knob, a flat bottom and a ring foot. As a daily life article of the nobility, it is polished, gilded and carved in designs.

Preserved in Tibet Museum

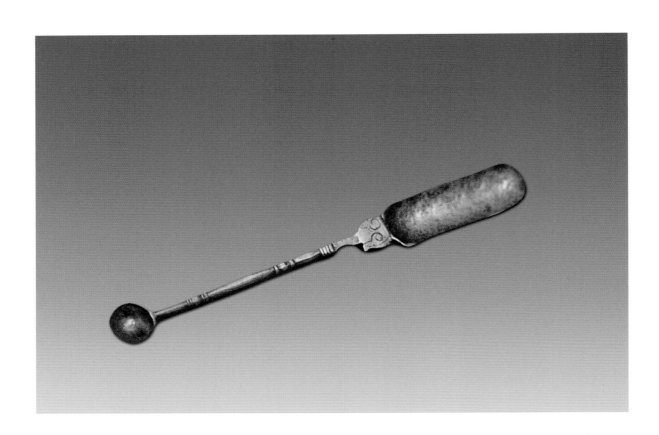

蒙医药勺

银质

长 20.5 厘米

Mongolian Medicine Spoon

Silver

Length 20.5 cm

传世品。此勺一端为圆勺，一端为长勺，用以取用不同剂量的药物。内蒙古阿拉善左旗征集。

北京中医药大学中医药博物馆藏

The spoon is handed down from ancient times. It has a round spoon at one end and a long deep spoon at the other. Both were used as tools for taking out and measuring medicinal powders. It was collected in Alxa Left Banner, Inner Mongolia Autonomous Region.

Preserved in The Museum of Chinese Medicine, Beijing University of Chinese Medicine

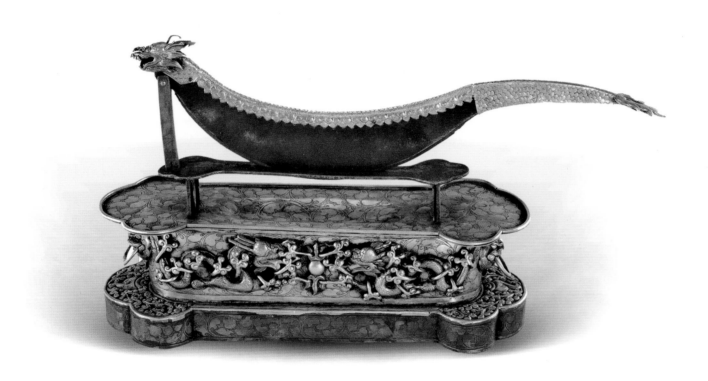

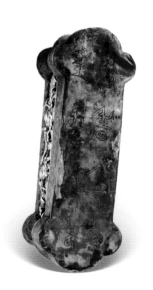

银质龙首铡刀

近现代

银质

长 42 厘米，高 25 厘米

用于切割药草。

内蒙古国际蒙医蒙药博物馆藏

Dragon Head-shaped Silver Chopper

Modern Times

Silver

Length 42 cm/ Height 25 cm

It was used to cut herb straw.

Preserved in Inner Mongolia International Mongolian

Medicine Museum

银质药碾

近现代

银质

通长 42.5 厘米，高 15 厘米

用于碾药。

内蒙古国际蒙医蒙药博物馆藏

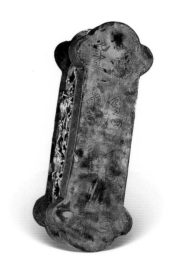

Silver Medicine Mill

Modern Times

Silver

Length 42.5 cm/ Height 15 cm

It was used to crush medicine into powder.

Preserved in Inner Mongolia International

Mongolian Medicine Museum

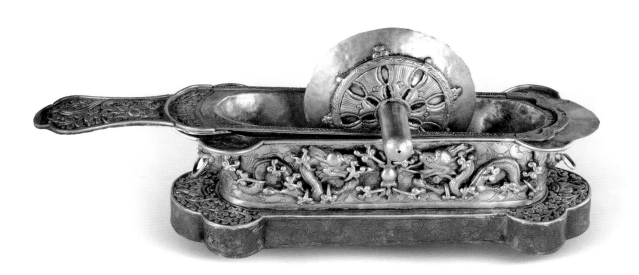

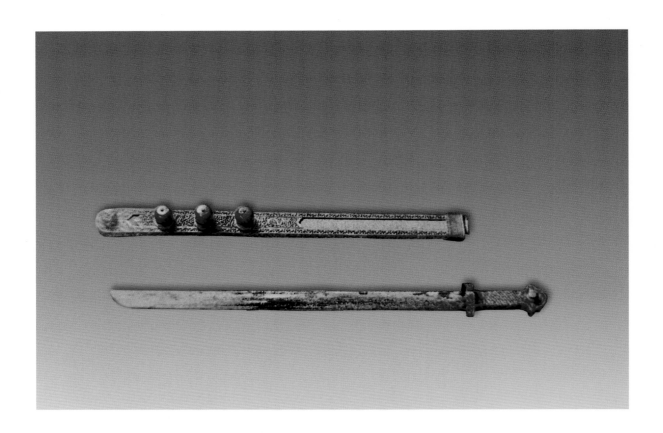

藏用腰刀

清

刀长 70.5 厘米

鞘长 63 厘米

Tibetan Broadsword

Qing Dynasty

Knife: Length 70.5 cm

Scabbard: Length 63 cm

作为砍劈器械的刀，在清代有长柄、短柄之
分。这一藏用腰刀，刃部锋利，直柄，有鞘，
为一藏族所用短柄刀。四川省甘孜藏族自治
州征集。

In the Qing Dynasty, broadswords were
classified into two types according to the length
of their handles—long handle broadswords and
short handle broadswords. This short straight
handle broadsword, with a sharp edge and a
scabbard, was used for chopping by Tibetans.
It was collected in Ganzi Tibetan Autonomous
Prefecture, Sichuan Province.

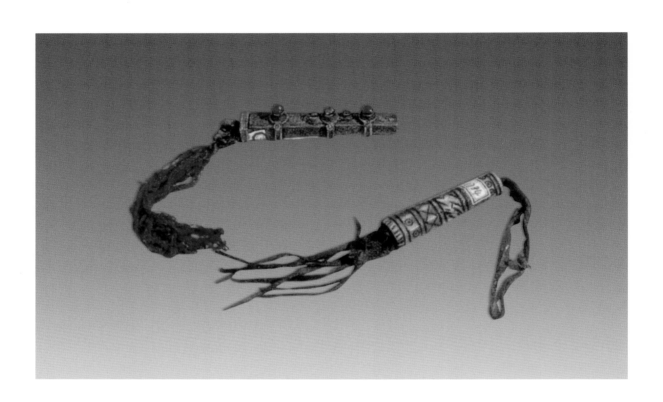

针线盒

20 世纪初

银质、骨质

银质长 12.5 厘米

骨质长 8.5 厘米

Workbox

Early 20th Century

Silver, Bone

Silver part: Length 12.5 cm

Bone part: Length 8.5 cm

棱柱形，刻有"O""X"等纹饰，镶绿松石和红珊瑚。

西藏博物馆藏

The prismatic workbox is carved with "O", "X" –shaped patterns, and is inlaid with calaite and red coral.

Preserved in Tibet Museum

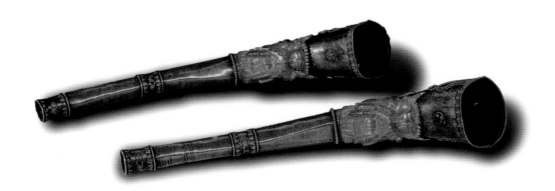

镶金银质仿胫骨号

清

镶金银质

口径 6.2 厘米，长 48 厘米

Gold-Inlaid Shinbone-Shaped Silver Horns

Qing Dynasty

Silver

Mouth Diameter 6.2 cm/ Length 48 cm

外形如同人的小腿骨，口沿及号筒连接处镶嵌有宝石、镶金质兽首。胫骨号是藏传密宗的法器之一，也是一种乐器，常成对使用。

西藏博物馆藏

The shape of these horns is similar to the human shinbone. Gems and gold animal-shaped heads are inlaid around the mouth as well as the joint of the horns. Shinbone-shaped silver horns are used either as ritual items of Tibetan Esoteric Buddhism or the musical instrument, and they are usually used in pairs.

Preserved in Tibet Museum

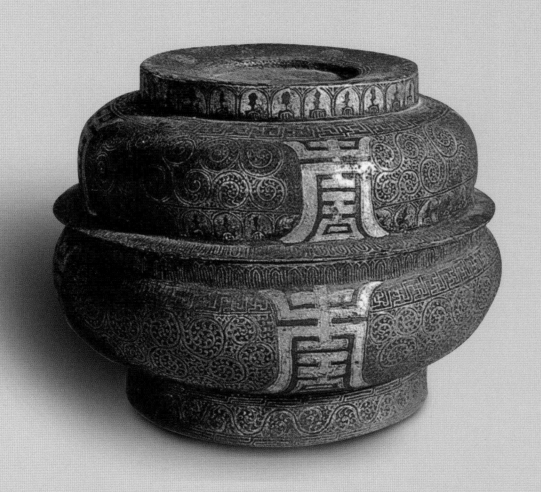

错金银质糌粑盒

20 世纪

错金银质

口径 19.7 厘米，底径 14.4 厘米，高 16.4 厘米

子母口，外撇，鼓腹，平底，圈足，器身布云纹，盖与盒形近，平钮，钮边缘饰宝塔纹一周。盖与器身上错金"万"字。

西藏博物馆藏

Gold-inlaid Silver Zanba Hamper

20th Century

Silver

Mouth Diameter 19.7 cm/ Bottom Diameter 14.4 cm/ Height 16.4 cm

The hamper has a snap–lid, a bulging belly, a flat Bottom, and a ring foot. Its body is decorated with cloud patterns. Similarly shaped as the body, the flat-knobbed cover is decorated with a circle of pagoda patterns. Chinese characters "Wan" are gilded on both the cover and body.

Preserved in Tibet Museum

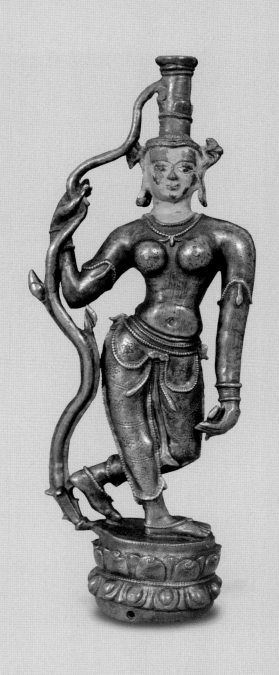

合金铜供养女烛台

12—13 世纪

合金铜

宽 9 厘米，高 21.8 厘米

供养女形象烛台，供器，常见于藏传佛教寺院里。

西藏博物馆藏

Female-donor-shaped Alloy Copper Candelabrum

12th -13th Century

Alloy Copper

Width 9 cm/ Height 21.8 cm

The female-donor-shaped candelabrum was used for the sacrificial ceremony. It is popular in Tibetan Buddhist temples.

Preserved in Tibet Museum

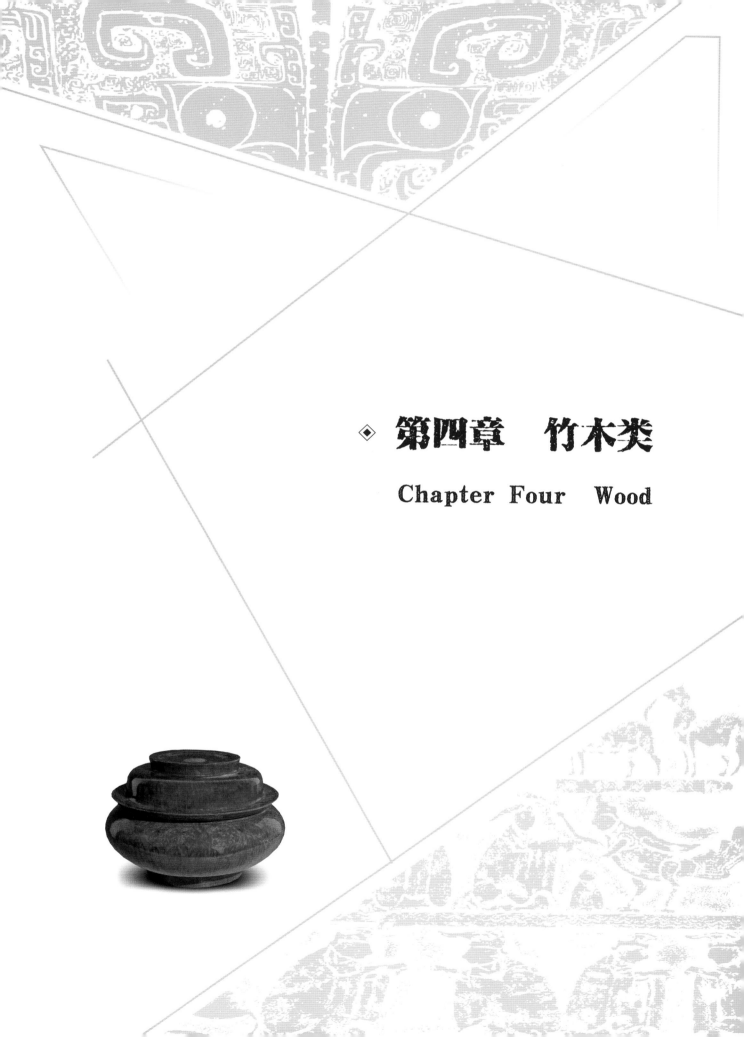

◇ 第四章　竹木类

Chapter Four　Wood

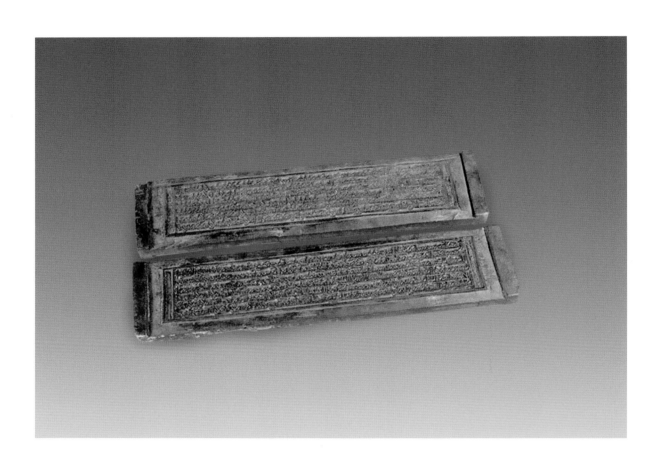

藏医书《祖先口述》印版

清

木质

长 34.5 厘米，宽 7.5 厘米

Printing Plates of Tibetan Medical Book *Zu Xian Kou Shu* (Ancestors' Dictation)

Qing Dynasty

Wood

Length 34.5 cm/ Width 7.5 cm

藏医著作《祖先口述》之木刻板。藏医学著作，又译为《美布协隆》，16 世纪藏医学家舒卡·洛珠给布著。该书主要对《四部医典》中的三部：《根本医典》《论说医典》《后续医典》做了最详尽的注释。

中国医史博物馆藏

This was the printing plate of a Tibetan medical book *Zu Xian Kou Shu* (Ancestors' Dictation). As a classic of Tibetan medicine, the book was written by the famous Tibetan medical scientist, Shuka Luozhugeibu. It was also translated into Chinese as *Mei Bu Xie Long*. It had given the most detailed annotation to three volumes of *The Four Medical Tantras*: *The Root Tantra, Argumentation Tantra, and Verification Tantra.* Preserved in Chinese Medical History Museum

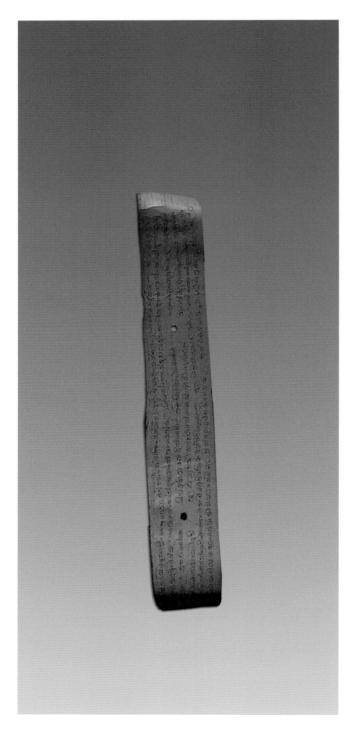

西藏喇嘛驱鬼治病符

清

树木皮

长 40 厘米，宽 5.5 厘米，厚 0.1 厘米

Tibetan Lama Amulet

Qing Dynasty

Bark

Length 40 cm/ Width 5.5 cm/ Thickness 0.1 cm

藏医用品之一，用藏文书写于植物叶上，内容是喇嘛驱鬼治病的咒语。长带形，用于医事活动。基本完好，折痕较重，表面有污迹。1953 年入藏。

中华医学会 / 上海中医药大学医史博物馆藏

Preserved as a Tibetan medical tool, the amulet was used for expelling evil spirits and curing diseases in medical practices by Tibetan lama. It is generally written in Tibetan on leaves. Except for some surface stains and heavy creases, it is still well preserved. It was collected in 1953. Preserved in Chinese Medical Association/ Museum of Chinese Medicine, Shanghai University of Traditional Chinese Medicine

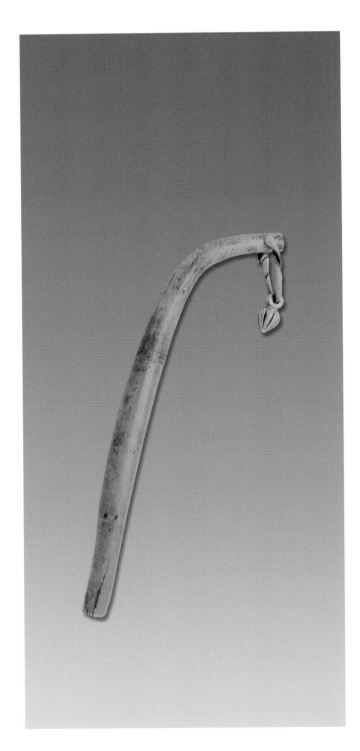

链锤布鲁

清

木质

通长 57.5 厘米

Hammer Bulu

Qing Dynasty

Wood

Length 57.5 cm

前部稍弯曲，似手杖形，首端有一孔，穿皮条连接一心状铜锤。"布鲁"为蒙语投掷之意，早在1300多年前就已成为游牧民族打猎和对敌战争的武器。后来逐渐演化成为远距离投掷项目用的运动器械。用布鲁投掷讲究距离远和目标准确，有利于增强臂力，锻炼力量、速度、灵敏及准确的目测能力。

内蒙古博物院藏

In the bent upper part of the cane-like bulu is a hole through which a leather belt is connected with a heart-shaped copper hammer. Bulu, meaning throwing in Mongolian, was used as a weapon for hunting as well as fighting against enemies by nomads as early as 1,300 years ago. Later on, it has gradually evolved into a sports equipment for long-distance throwing events. The game maximizes long-distance throwing and target accuracy and is beneficial to the enhancing of muscles, physical power, speed, sensitivity and accuracy of visual inspection ability.

Preserved in Inner Mongolia Museum

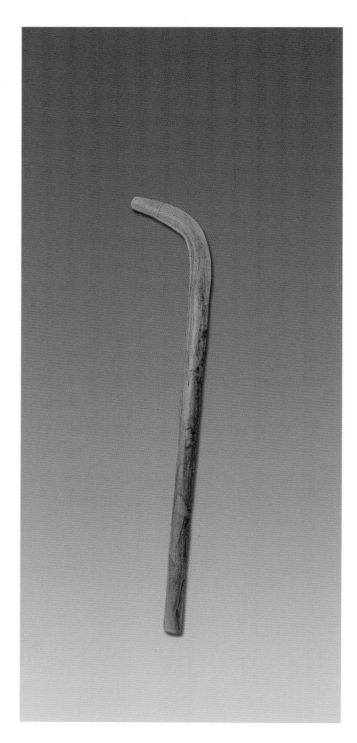

包铁布鲁

清

木质

通长 59 厘米

Iron-covered Bulu

Qing Dynasty

Wood

Length 59 cm

末端稍弯曲，首部包铁皮。护牧狩猎和远距
离投掷运动项目用的主要器械。

内蒙古博物院藏

The bottom part is slightly bent with its top
covered with iron sheet. It was the main
instrument for protecting the herd, hunting and
long-distance throwing events.
Preserved in Inner Mongolia Museum

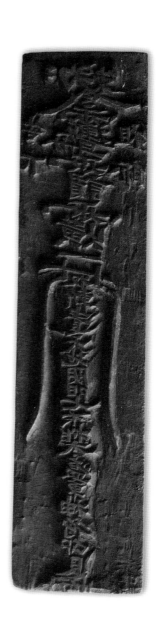

木刻符印版

清

木质

宽 6 厘米，高 37 厘米，厚 3.8 厘米

仫佬族驱邪符印版。罗城四把镇棉花村征集。

罗城仫佬族博物馆藏

Wooden Printing Board of Spells

Qing Dynasty

Wood

Width 6 cm/ Height 37 cm/ Thickness 3.8 cm

The Mulao printed exorcism spells with the printing board. It was collected at Mianhua Village, Siba Town, Luocheng Mulao Autonomous County.

Preserved in Luocheng Mulao Museum

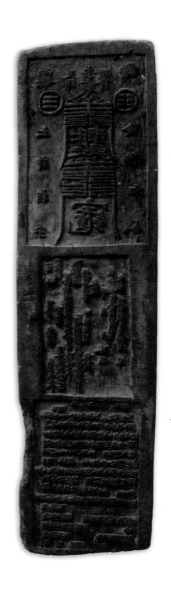
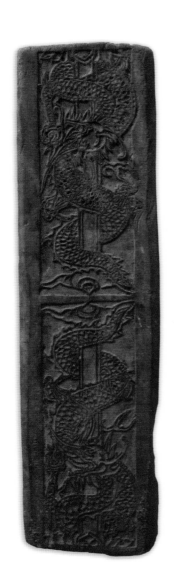

双面神龙纹法符木刻板

清

木质

宽 14 厘米，高 29 厘米，厚 4.6 厘米

仫佬族驱邪符木刻板。罗城四把镇新印村征集。

罗城仫佬族博物馆藏

Wooden Printing Board of Spells Engraved with Dragon Patterns on Both Sides

Qing Dynasty

Wood

Width 14 cm/ Height 29 cm/ Thickness 4.6 cm

The Mulao printed exorcism spells with the printing board. It was collected at Xinyin Village, Siba Town, Luocheng Mulao Autonomous County.

Preserved in Luocheng Mulao Museum

驱邪呵令木法器

清

木质

最长 20.5 厘米，最宽 4.2 厘米，厚 3.8 厘米

仫佬族驱邪用具。罗城东门镇桥头村征集。

罗城仫佬族博物馆藏

Wooden Magic Instrument with Exorcism Spells

Qing Dynasty

Wood

Maximum Length 20.5 cm/ Maximum Width
4.2 cm/ Thickness 3.8 cm

These were Mulao's exorcism ware. These were
collected at Qiaotou Village, Dongmen Town,
Luocheng Mulao Autonomous Count.

Preserved in Luocheng Mulao Museum

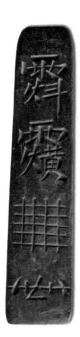

正面
Front

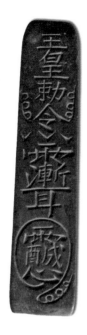

背面
Back

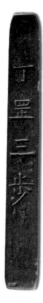

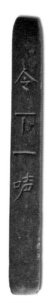

正面
Front

背面
Back

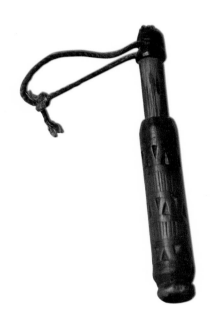

竹刻纹针筒

清

木质

长 13 厘米，直径 1.2 厘米

仡佬族用具。罗城东门镇大福村藏品。

吴桂文藏

Needle Holder with Bamboo Patterns

Qing Dynasty

Wood

Length 13 cm/ Diameter 2.1 cm

The holder was used by the Mulao. It is preserved at Dafu Village, Dongmen Town, Luocheng Mulao Autonomous County.

Collected by Wu Guiwen

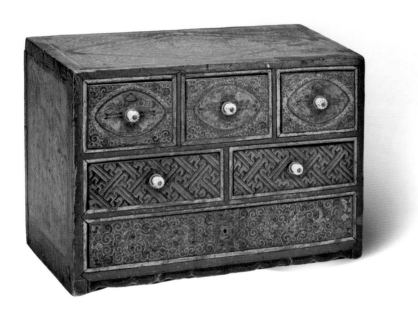

彩绘六屉木柜

清

木质

高 52 厘米

用于装药。

内蒙古博物院藏

Painted Six-drawer Cabinet

Qing Dynasty

Wood

Height 52 cm

It was used to store medicine.

Preserved in Inner Mongolia Museum

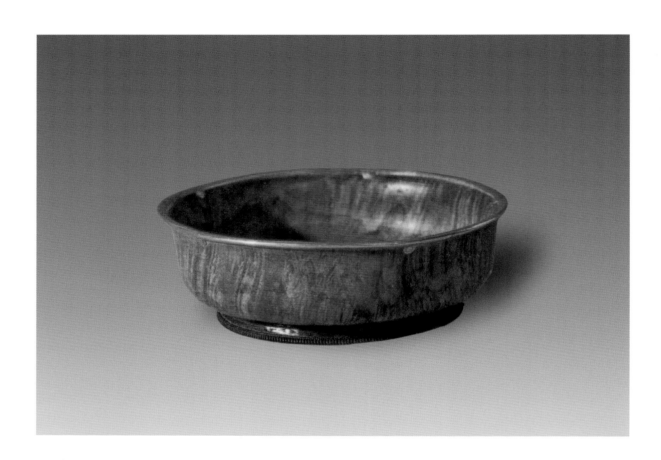

金扣木碗

19 世纪

木质，金扣

口径 13.5 厘米，底径 9.5 厘米，高 9.5 厘米

Gold-rimmed Wooden Bowl

19th century

Wood, Gold

Mouth Diameter 13.5 cm/ Bottom Diameter 9.5 cm/ Height 9.5 cm

敞口，口沿以金做箍，微外撇，平底，圈足。木碗是藏族、门巴族和珞巴族最喜欢的生活用具，也是民族工艺品之一。木碗不但具有不烫手、不烫嘴、不走味和保持温度等优点，而且不易打碎，轻便易带，很适合牧人游牧生活使用。

西藏博物馆藏

The gold-rimmed wooden bowl has an open mouth, a flat bottom, and a ring foot. It is not only the favorite life article but also handicraft article of the Tibetan nationality, the Moinba nationality and the Lhoba nationality. It can keep one's mouth and hands from being burnt, and preserve the flavor and the temperature of the food. It is also portable and breakage-proof, which makes it suitable for the nomadic life.

Preserved in Tibet Museum

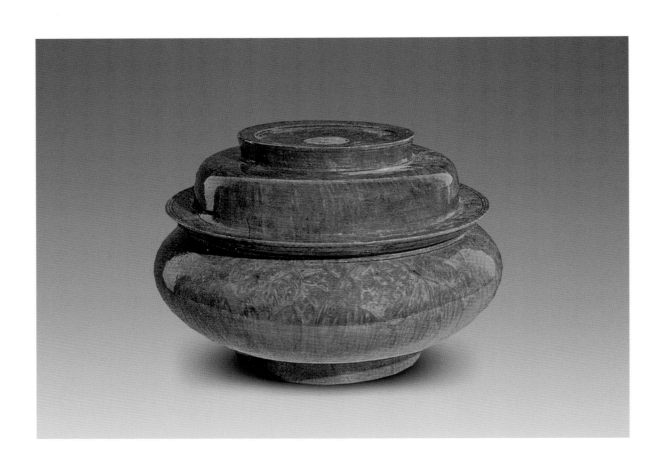

根瘤木质糌粑盒

20 世纪

木质

口径 23.7 厘米，最大直径 31.5 厘米，高 19.3 厘米

Wood-Nodule Made Zanba Hamper

20th Century

Wood

Mouth Diameter 23.7 cm/ Maximum Diameter 31.5 cm/ Height 19.3 cm

广口，带盖，鼓腹。用于存放糌粑。糌粑是藏族特有的一种主食，流行于西藏、四川、青海、甘肃、云南等藏族聚居地区。藏族日常生活用品。

西藏博物馆藏

The hamper has a wide mouth, a lid, and a bulging body. It was used as a daily life article to store zanba which is the staple food of Tibetans and is popular in the Tibetan-inhabited areas of Tibet, Sichuan, Qinghai, Gansu and Yunnan.

Preserved in Tibet Museum

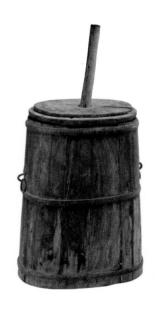

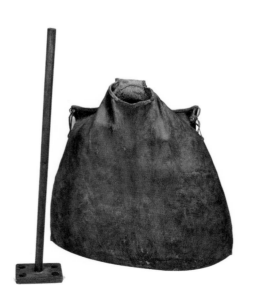

拼木酸奶扁桶

近现代

木质

高 44 厘米

用于蒙医饮食疗法。

内蒙古博物院藏

Flat Spliced Wooden Yoghourt Bucket

Modern Times

Wood

Height 44 cm

It was used in Mongolian diet therapy.

Preserved in Inner Mongolia Museum

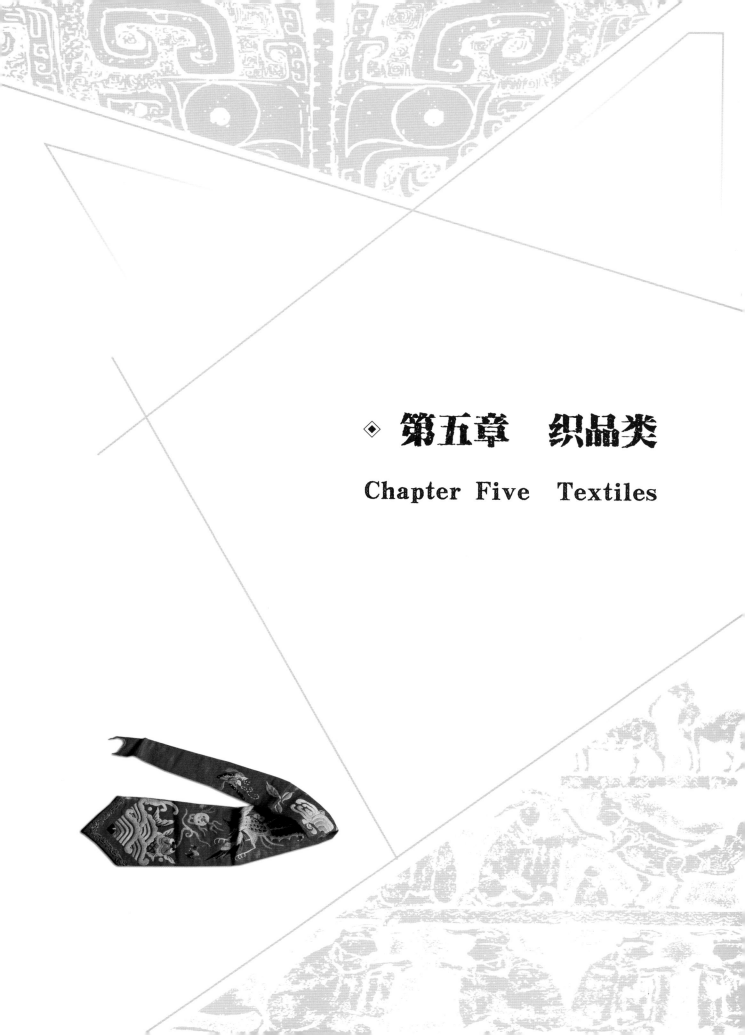

◈ 第五章　织品类

Chapter Five　Textiles

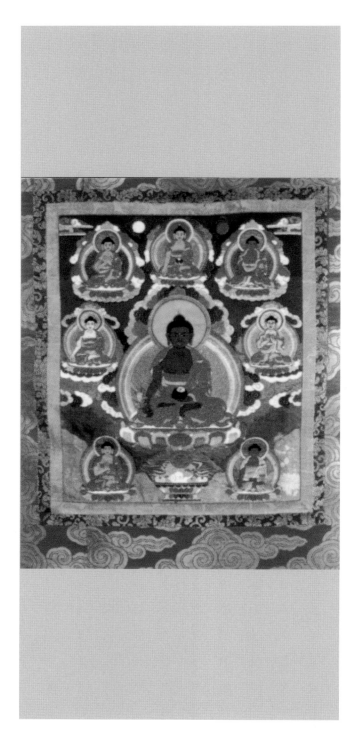

八大药师佛像唐卡

清

堆绣

长 84.5 厘米，宽 68.3 厘米

Thangka of Eight Medicine Buddhas

Qing Dynasty

Barbola

Length 84.5 cm/ Width 68.3 cm

药师佛，又作"药师如来""药师琉璃光如来"，为东方净琉璃世界之教主。化导众生，拔除生死之疾病。作为藏族文化中一种独具特色的绘画艺术形式的唐卡，融入了苗族堆绣的制作工艺中。

西藏博物馆藏

Medicine Buddha, who is also called Medicine Guru Buddha or Medicine Bhaishajyaguru, is the hierarch of the East Bhaishajyaguru. Medicine Buddha can guide the creatures and avert fatal diseases. As a unique artistic form of drawing in Tibetan culture, this thangka has also borrowed the manufacturing techniques of barbola from the Miao nationality.

Preserved in Tibet Museum

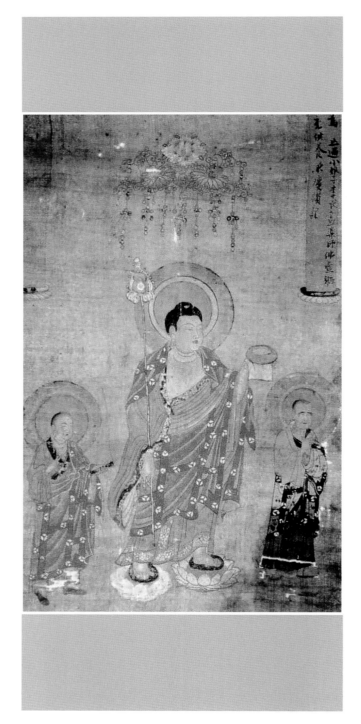

药师佛画像

唐

绢绸画

Portrait of Medicine Buddha

Tang Dynasty

Silk

半侧面行走像，上方有花饰，右上方有"奉为止过小娘子李氏画药师佛一躯，永供充养，兼庆赞记"等题词，其旁有两位僧人陪伴，可能为阿难陀和大迦叶佛。据甘肃敦煌千佛洞复制。

甘肃敦煌千佛洞藏

The Buddha is walking in a half profile image. The upper part of the picture is decorated with flowers, and on the upper right part are inscriptions saying that "the Medicine Buddha's portrait is drawn for my deceased young wife nee Li, hoping it could support her forever. And the portrait is also a token of expressing my greatest appreciation to Buddha." Standing beside the Buddha are two Buddhist monks who might be the Venerable Ananda and Kashyapa Buddha. It was copied from the Thousand-Buddha Cave in the Mogao Grottoes in Dunhuang, Gansu Province.

Preserved in the Thousand-Buddha Cave in Dunhuang, Gansu Province

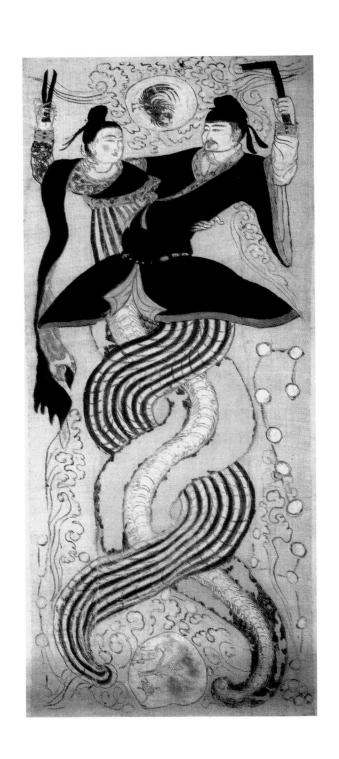

伏羲女娲交尾图

唐

绢质

纵 220 厘米，横 116.5 厘米

伏羲女娲是中国古代传说中的人类始祖。以白、红、黄、黑四色描绘，人首蛇身。伏羲在左，左手执矩，教授人们生活和生产的法度。女娲在右，右手执规，教化人们婚嫁与道德规范的准则或常理。二者彼此环抱，人首蛇身，蛇尾交缠，头上绘日，尾间绘月，周围绘满星辰。构图奇特，寓意深刻。这种图像常见于新疆吐鲁番地区的夫妻合葬墓，多用木钉钉在墓顶上，少数则折叠包好放在死者身旁。

新疆维吾尔自治区博物馆藏

Fuxi and Nüwa's Mating Picture

Tang Dynasty

Silk

Length 220 cm/ Width 116.5 cm

Fuxi and Nüwa are the ancestors of ancient Chinese legends. In the picture, they are painted in the four colours of white, red, yellow and black, with human heads and snake bodies. Fuxi is in the left, with his left hand holding the moment, teaching people the laws of life and production. Nüwa is in the right with her right hand holding a rule, educating people about marriage and moral norms or common sense. With human heads and snake bodies, they embrace each other and their tails intertwine. The sun is painted on their head, whereas the moon is painted on their tails and stars are painted around them. The picture has a particular composition and profound implications. This image is common in the couples burial tombs in Xinjiang Turpan area, as most of the pictures of this kind are nailed on top of the tomb with dowels, and a few of them would be folded and put beside the dead.

Preserved in Xinjiang Uygur Autonomous Region Museum

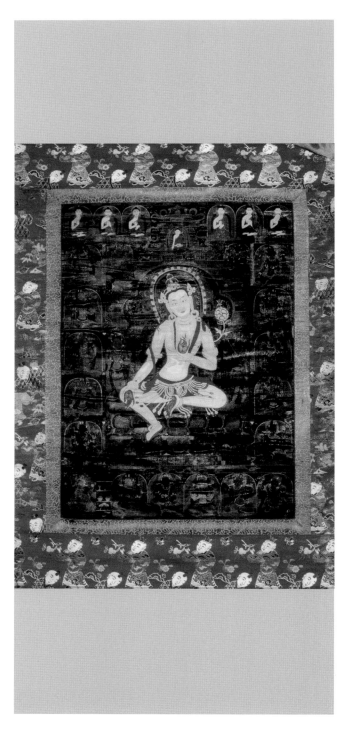

救八难度母像唐卡

明

布画

长 60 厘米，宽 44 厘米

Thangka of Averting Tara Eight Calamities

Ming Dynasty

Fabric

Length 60 cm/ Width 44 cm

彩绘，描金。绿度母，又称"救八难度母"，
能解除狮难（傲慢）、象难（愚痴）、火难（嗔
恚）、蛇难（嫉妒）、贼难（邪见）、牢狱难（吝
啬）、非人难（疑惑）及水难等八种苦难。

西藏博物馆藏

This colored drawing is traced in gold. In
Tibetan Buddhism, Tara, who is also called
Eight Calamities Averting Tara, can avert
the following eight calamities: lion calamity
(arrogance), elephant calamity (imbecility), fire
calamity (anger), snake calamity (jealousy),
thief calamity (deviant intentions), prison
calamity (parsimony), nonhuman calamity
(doubt) and water calamity.

Preserved in Tibet Museum

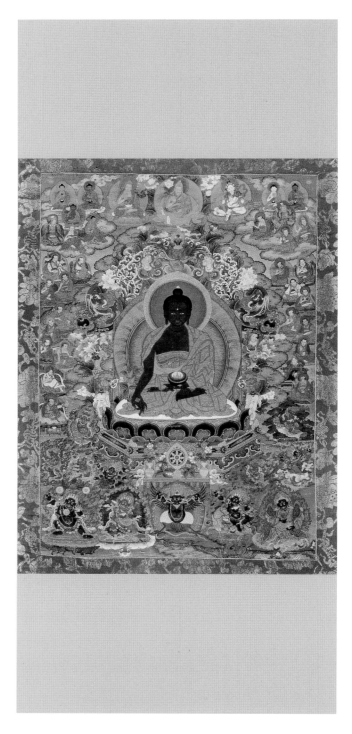

藏医药师承图

清

布画

长 68 厘米，宽 47 厘米

Picture of Tibetan Medicine Buddha Succession

Qing Dynasty

Fabric

Length 68 cm/ Width 47 cm

《四部医典》系列彩色挂图之一，图示公元5世纪至8世纪的藏医学家，中间为药师佛像。

布达拉宫藏

This is one of the series of pictures of *Si Bu Yi Dian* (The Four Medical Tantras). The figures shown in the picture are Tibetan medical scientists during the 5th century through the 8th century. Right in the middle of the picture is the Medicine Buddha.

Preserved in the Potala Palace

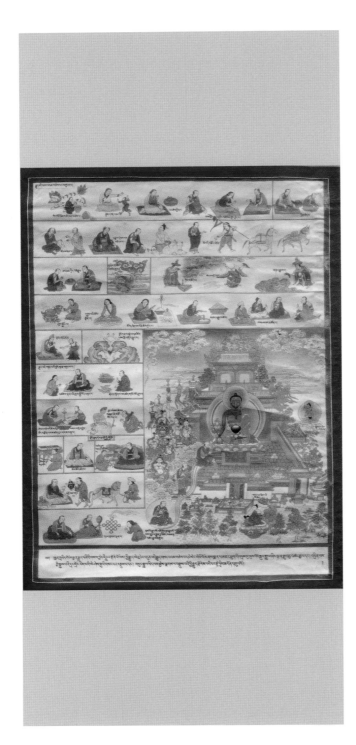

《四部医典》总结图谱唐卡

清

布画

长 104 厘米，宽 73 厘米

Thangka of *Si Bu Yi Dian* (The Four Medical Tantras Outline)

Qing Dynasty

Fabric

Length 104 cm/ Width 73 cm

着色。《四部医典》是一部藏医学经典著作，藏文原名《华丹据悉》。由"根本部""论说部""秘诀部""后读部"四部分组成，全书共156章，24万余字。

西藏博物馆藏

The color is put on the finished drawing. The *Si Bu Yi Dian* (*Hua Dan Ju Xi* in Tibetan) is a classic work of Tibetan medicine. It consists of four volumes—Root Tantra, Argumentation Tantra, Secret Tantra and Verification Tantra. It has 156 chapters with more than 240,000 characters.

Preserved in Tibet Museum

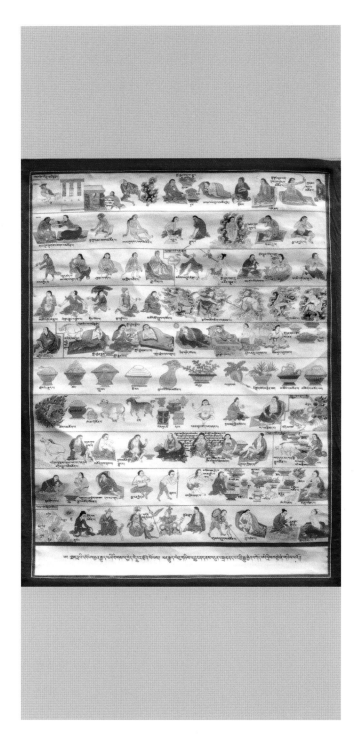

隆赤巴培根病因分析图唐卡

清

布画

长 104 厘米，宽 73 厘米

Thangka of Pathological Analysis by Long, Chiba and Peigen Schools

Qing Dynasty

Fabric

Length 104 cm/ Width 73 cm

着色。"隆""赤巴""培根"是藏医学基本理论的三个概念，是人体原理的基本要素。此唐卡以图像的形式分析"隆""赤巴""培根"的病因。

西藏博物馆藏

The color is put on the finished drawing. The three theories of Long, Chiba and Peigen are both the basic concepts of the traditional Tibetan medicine and fundamental elements of the principles for human body analysis. This thangka shows how pathologcal analyses are carried out in the form of images.

Preserved in Tibet Museum

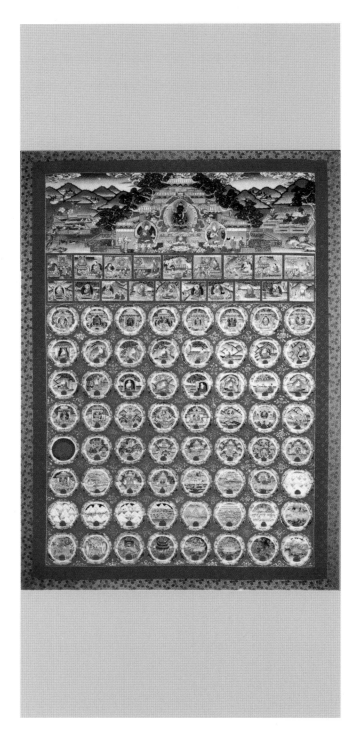

次第道游戏图唐卡

清末

布画

长 118.4 厘米，宽 78.3 厘米

Thangka of Graduated Path Game Picture

Late Qing Dynasty

Fabric

Length 118.4 cm/ Width 78.3 cm

彩绘，描金。本唐卡以游戏的图案展示次第
道修炼的过程。次第道是藏传佛教的修炼功
法之一，能使人的躯体等变为无有障害之轮，
象征因果无别。

西藏博物馆藏

This colored drawing is traced in gold. It
displays the process of playing the Graduated
Path Game. The game is one of the Tibetan
Buddhist doctrines and is believed to turn the
human body into a wheel free from being hurt,
which symbolizes that there is no difference
between cause and effect.

Preserved in Tibet Museum

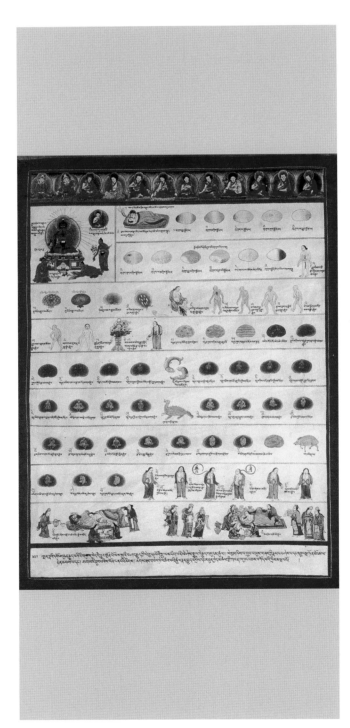

藏医胚胎发育图

清

亚麻布画

Tibetan Medical Picture of Embryonic Development

Qing Dynasty

Linen

据《四部医典》内容绘画。藏医认为人类胚胎发育须经鱼期、龟期、猪期三个阶段。本图即按照上述认识，形象而生动地描绘了人体胚胎发育的各个阶段。

西藏自治区藏医药研究院藏

The picture was drawn in accordance with *Si Bu Yi Dian* (The Four Medical Tantras). In Tibetan medicine, it is believed that the development of human embryo experiences three stages—fish stage, turtle stage and pig stage. And this picture is a vivid description of each stage of human embryo development Bottomd on the above belief.

Preserved in Tibet Autonomous Region Institute of Tibetan Medicine

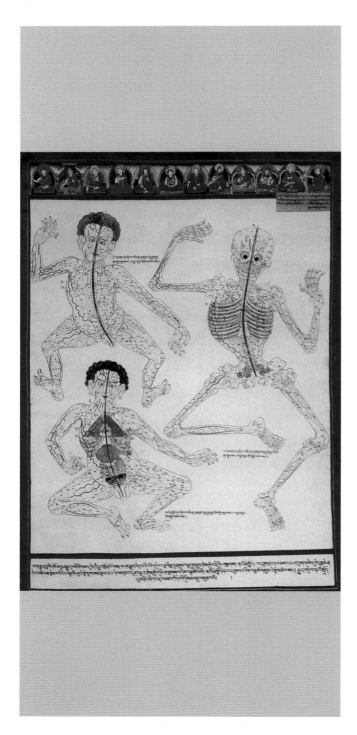

藏医脉络图

清

亚麻布画

长 103 厘米，宽 72 厘米

Tibetan Medical Picture of Mailuo

Qing Dynasty

Linen

Length 103 cm/ Width 72 cm

藏医把人体内的脉络分为白脉和黑脉，前者
为神经，后者为血管。本图据《四部医典》
绘制，用不同颜色的数字标明内脏脉、骨骼
脉、皮肉间脉络的部位和区间。

西藏自治区藏医药研究院藏

In Tibetan medicine, Mailuo is divided into two
types of White and Black ones, and the former
refers to nerves while the latter blood vessels.
Drawn in accordance with *Si Bu Yi Dian* (The
Four Medical Tantras), the picture uses different
colored numbers to indicate different Mailuo of
internal organs, skeleton and Mailuo between
parts and the whole.
Preserved in Tibet Autonomous Region Institute
of Tibetan Medicine

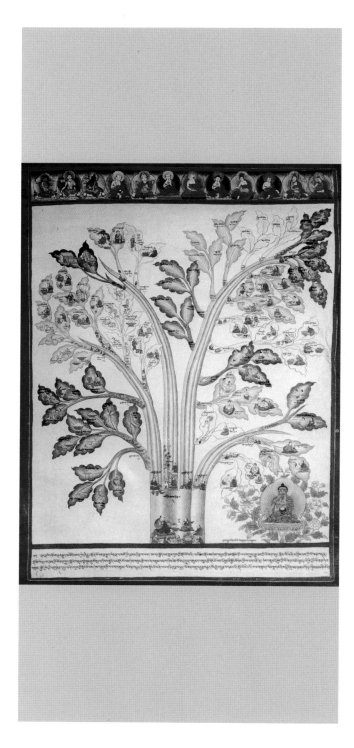

藏医食行药察图

清

亚麻布画

长 103 厘米，宽 72 厘米

Tibetan Medical Observation Picture on Food and Behavior

Qing Dynasty

Linen

Length 103 cm/ Width 72 cm

公元 17 世纪，弟斯桑结嘉措在前人注释基础上编成《四部医典大注蓝琉璃》，书中认为医生观察疾病，首先要从病人的食物、行为了解病因，辨证论治。后召集全区名画家，实际观察和收集药物标本，于公元 1704 年绘制 79 幅彩色医药学挂图。本图为其中之一，图中把上述主张形象地画成 4 棵大树，以树叶说明食行药察的情节，并附有文字说明。

西藏自治区藏医药研究院藏

Si Bu Yi Dian Da Zhu Lan Liu Li (The Blue Beryl), a new commentary on *Si Bu Yi Dian* (The Four Medical Tantras), was compiled by Desi Sangye Gyatso in the 17th century who believed that doctors were supposed to learn the causes of disease from the patients' food and behavior so that they could make treatment Bottomd on syndrome differentiation. He invited all the celebrated painters in Tibet to observe and collect medicine specimen and finally drew 79 colorized medical wall charts in 1704. This picture is just one of them. It vividly embodies the above belief in four trees, each of whose leaves stands for a plot for doctors to observe the patient's food and behavior. Captions are also available.

Preserved in Tibet Autonomous Region Institute of Tibetan Medicine

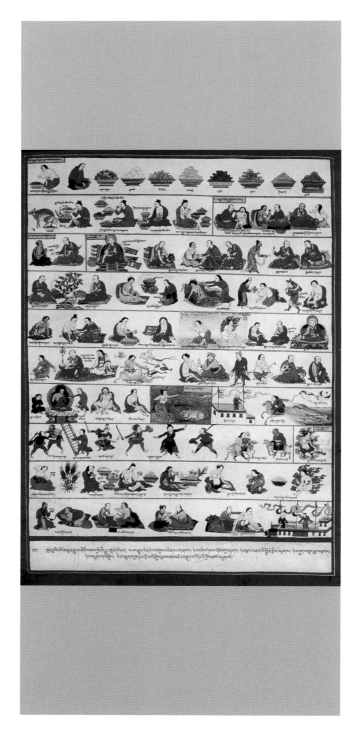

藏医诊治图

清

亚麻布画

长 103 厘米，宽 72 厘米

Picture of Tibetan Diagnosis and Treatment

Qing Dynasty

Linen

Length 103 cm/ Width 72 cm

据《四部医典》绘画。藏医诊病主要通过问诊、触诊（切脉）、望诊，诊察病人五官、躯体、排泄物、血、脉、体温、疼痛等的变化与情况，分析判断"隆"（气）、"赤巴"（火）、"培根"（水与土）的有余、不足，以确定疾病的部位、性质等，据此确立治疗原则和方法。本图形象地描绘了藏医诊疗疾病的理论和方法。

西藏自治区藏医药研究院藏

The picture was drawn in accordance with *Si Bu Yi Dian* (The Four Medical Tantras). By means of inquiry, palpation and observation, Tibetan doctors examine the changes of the patients' facial features, body, excrement, blood, veins, body temperature and pain so as to analyze whether "Long (qi), Chiba (fire) and Peigen (water and earth)" are normal and then identify the location and nature of disease, on which treatment principles and methods will be applied.The picture vividly depicts the theories and methods of Tibetan Medicine for diaghosing and treating diseases.

Preserved in Tibet Autonomous Region Institute of Tibetan Medicine

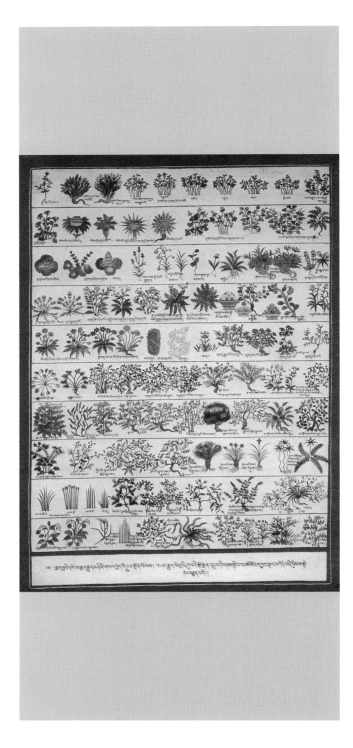

藏医植物药图

清

亚麻布画

长 103 厘米，宽 72 厘米

Picture of Tibetan Medical Herbs

Qing Dynasty

Linen

Length 103 cm/ Width 72 cm

据《四部医典》绘制。藏药品种繁多，包括植物药、矿物药、动物药，尤以植物药的应用更为广泛。图为藏医部分植物药的彩绘图。

西藏自治区藏医药研究院藏

The picture was drawn in accordance with *Si Bu Yi Dian* (The Four Medical Tantras). There are a great variety of Tibetan medicines, which include herbs, mineral drugs and animal drugs. In particular, herbs are extensively applied. The colored picture just contains parts of Tibetan medical herbs.

Preserved in Tibet Autonomous Region Institute of Tibetan Medicine

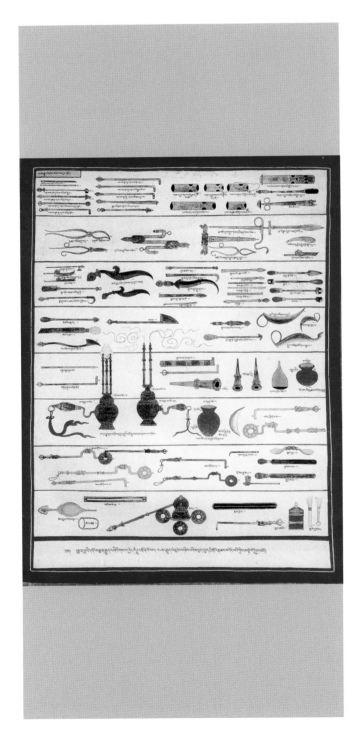

藏医医疗器械图

清

亚麻布画

长 103 厘米，宽 72 厘米

Picture of Tibetan Medical Apparatus

Qing Dynasty

Linen

Length 103 cm/ Width 72 cm

据《四部医典》绘制。收绘的藏医医疗器械约 90 种，包括诊断器械、外科手术器械及治疗器具，如肛门镜、外科手术刀、钳、镊、锯、钩、环钻、吸入器具及艾灸器具等，反映出藏医学医疗技术已达到较高水平。

西藏自治区藏医药研究院藏

Drawn in accordance with *Si Bu Yi Dian* (The Four Medical Tantras), the picture shows about 90 kinds of medical apparatus, including diagnostic apparatus, surgical apparatus and therapeutic apparatus such as anoscope, scalpels, clamps, forceps, saws, hooks, trephines, suction devices, moxibustion apparatuses and so on, which shows that Tibetan medical technology has reached a higher level.

Preserved in Tibet Autonomous Region Institute of Tibetan Medicine

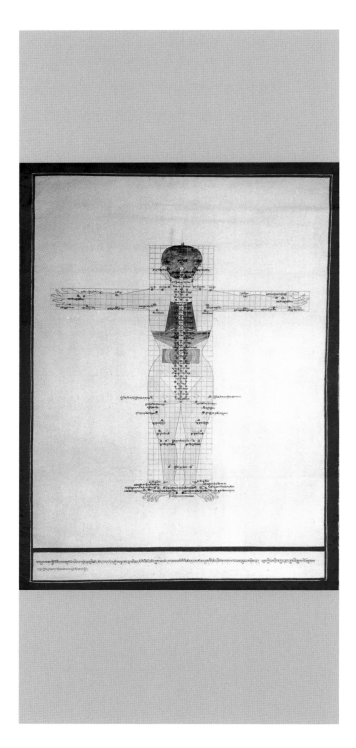

藏医穴位图

清

亚麻布画

长 103 厘米，宽 72 厘米

Picture of Tibetan Acupuncture Points

Qing Dynasty

Linen

Length 103 cm/ Width 72 cm

据《四部医典》绘画。藏医很重视放血、拔火罐、火灸等疗法，而且严格要求按一定的穴位进行。藏医穴位理论独具特色，有可放血的穴位，有拔火罐、火灸穴位，其中后两者与中医针灸穴位有相似之处。

西藏自治区藏医药研究院藏

The picture was drawn in accordance with *Si Bu Yi Dian* (The Four Medical Tantras). Tibetan doctors attach great importance to therapies of blood-letting, cupping, and fire moxibustion and observe them strictly on certain acupuncture points. The theory of Tibetan acupuncture points has unique features in that it has acupuncture points respectively for blood-letting, cupping and fire moxibustion, among which the last two have similarities to traditional Chinese medicine acupuncture points.

Preserved in Tibet Autonomous Region Institute of Tibetan Medicine

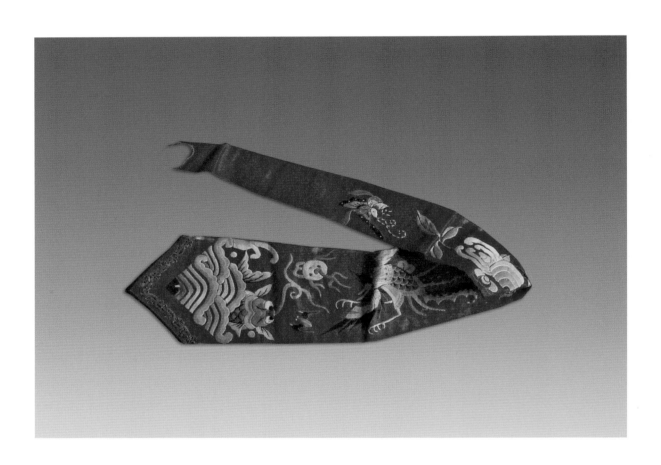

医病符

清

丝绵质

通长 78 厘米，宽 11 厘米

Amulet

Qing Dynasty

Silk, Cotton

Length 78 cm/ Width 11 cm

正面为丝织，背面棉织。正面绣有碧波赤日、鸟兽花卉等巫术图案，色彩鲜艳，构图有致。带形，为神符用品。喇嘛寺所用镇邪避灾、巫术医病之用品。1958年入藏。

中华医学会／上海中医药大学医史博物馆藏

This ribbon-shaped amulet has a silk front side and a cotton back side. On the front side are embroidered colorful and well-organized designs of green waves, a red sun, animals and flowers of magic power. It was mainly utilized for expelling evil spirits, avoiding disasters and curing diseases by lamasery. It was collected in 1958.

Preserved in Chinese Medical Association/ Museum of Chinese Medicine, Shanghai University of Traditional Chinese Medicine

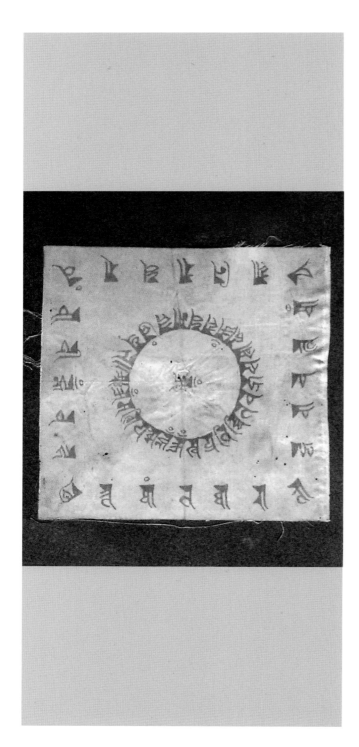

喇嘛寺医病符

清

丝织品

长 7.5 厘米，宽 7 厘米

Lamasery Amulet

Qing Dynasty

Silk Fabric

Length 7.5 cm/ Width 7 cm

方形，白色丝织品印红色佛经文字、粘贴于
蓝色硬板纸上。据背后所附纸条注，该藏是
蒙古喇嘛寺驱鬼医病咒条，出自山西太行山
外，蒙古境内最高山顶上的喇嘛寺内。详情
待考。辟邪用品。保存基本完好，丝织泛黄。

中华医学会 / 上海中医药大学医史博物馆藏

This square amulet is a kind of white silk
fabric with red Buddhist texts sticked to a blue
cardboard. According to the note attached to
its back, it was used for expelling evil spirits
and curing diseases by Mongolian lamasery. It
was collected from the lamasery on the highest
mountain in the Inner Mongolia Autonomous
Region, which is to the north of Taihang
Mountain in Shanxi Province. But more
information need be studied. Except for the
yellowish silk, it is still well preserved.

Preserved in Chinese Medical Association/
Museum of Chinese Medicine, Shanghai
University of Traditional Chinese Medicine

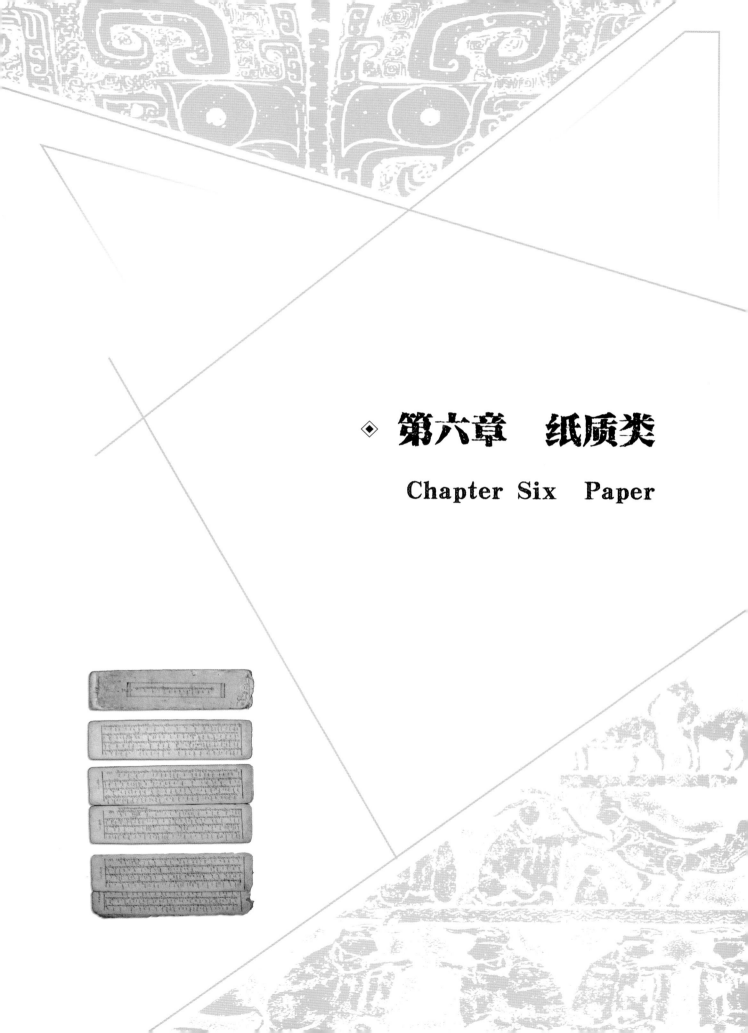

◈ 第六章　纸质类

Chapter Six　Paper

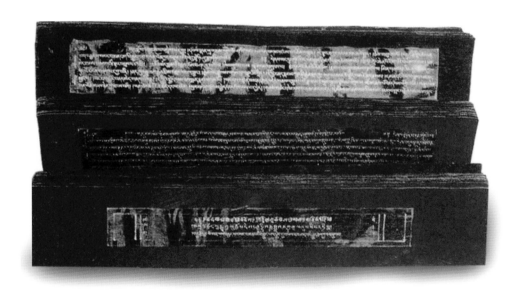

纯金粉写《四部医典》书影

清

清代藏医学家、书法家用纯金粉所书的抄写本，字迹经久不变，十分珍贵。藏医学经典著作《四部医典》系藏医学家宇妥·元丹贡布撰，约成书于公元 8 世纪。本书为集藏医学、中医学、印度医学于一体的巨著，对国内外均有广泛影响。现有汉文、蒙文及英文、俄文等多种文字的全译本流传。

布达拉宫藏

Manuscript of *Si Bu Yi Dian* Written in Pure Gold Powder

Qing Dynasty

This is the handwritten copy in pure gold powder by Tibetan medical scientists and calligraphers. It is really precious as the handwriting is still as new as it first appeared. The classical work *Si Bu Yi Dian* (The Four Medical Tantras) was compiled by Yutuo Yuandan Gongbu possibly in the 8th century. As a great work integrating Tibetan medicine, traditional Chinese medicine and Indian medicine, it still exerts extensive influence both at home and abroad. Up to now, it has cover-to-cover translations in Chinese, Mongolian, English, Russian and other languages.

Preserved in the Potala Palace

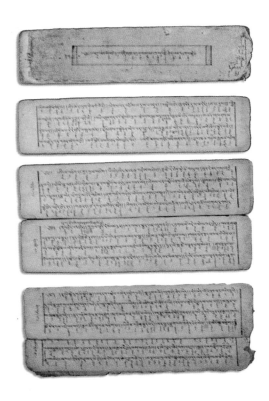

蒙藏文对照验方集

黄土纸

长 37 厘米，宽 9 厘米

手抄本。1978 年内蒙古扎旦召准国利喇嘛
所赠。

陕西医史博物馆藏

Collection of Proved Prescriptions in Both Mongolian and Tibetan

Ocher paper

Length 37 cm/ Width 9 cm

This handwritten copy was collected as a gift from a lama from the Inner Mongolia Autonomous Region in 1978.

Preserved in Shaanxi Museum of Medical History

第七章　其　他

Chapter Seven　Miscellanies

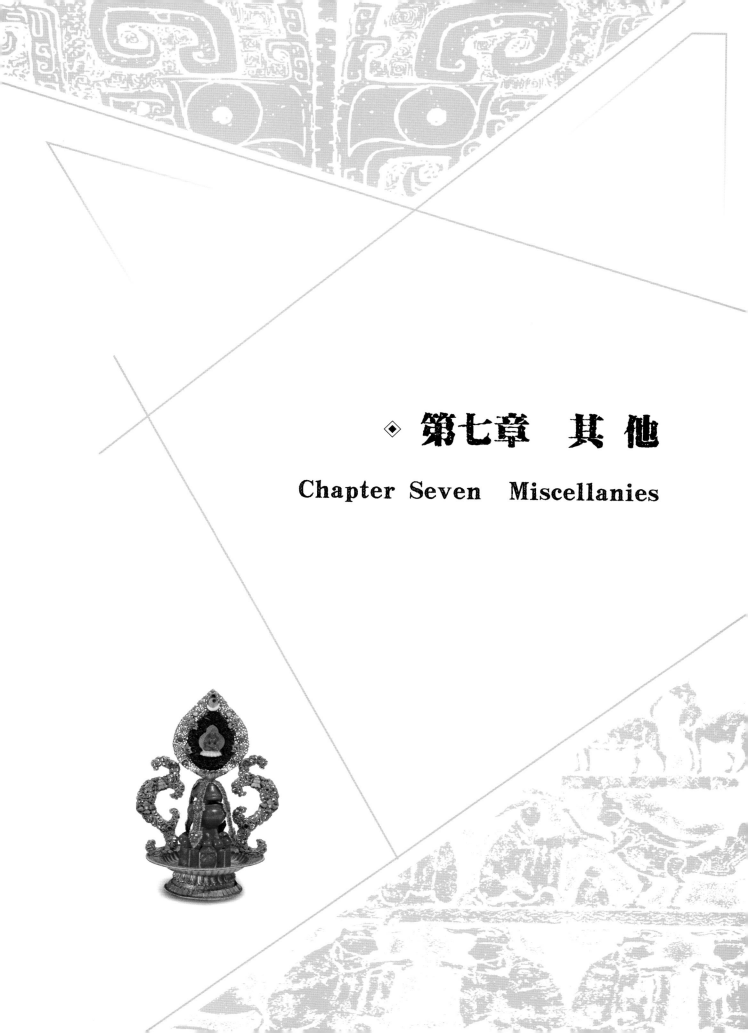

石质螭首

元

石质

长 91 厘米，宽 30 厘米，高 33 厘米

卷鼻，张口露齿，瞠目嗤鼻，昂首腆胸，螭首后上方有长方形凹槽，造型浑厚古朴。皇家蒙古族建筑的典型散水装置。河北省张北县馒头营乡元中都遗址出土。

元中都博物馆藏

Stone Chi Dragon Head

Yuan Dynasty

Stone

Length 91 cm/ Width 30 cm/ Height 33 cm

The Chi dragon holds its head up and throws out its chest, with nose curling up, teeth showing, and eyes glaring. On its rear is a rectangular groove. Simply and vigorously shaped, it was widely used for drainage in Mongolian royal courts. It was excavated at the former site of Yuanzhongdu Site at Mantouying Town, Zhangbei County, Hebei Province.

Preserved in Yuanzhongdu Museum

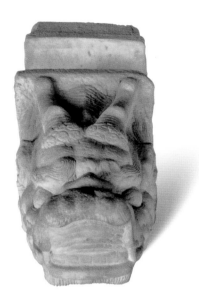

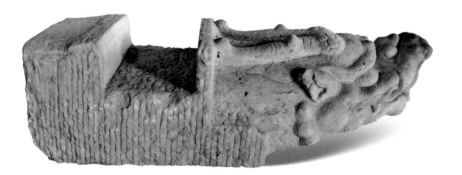

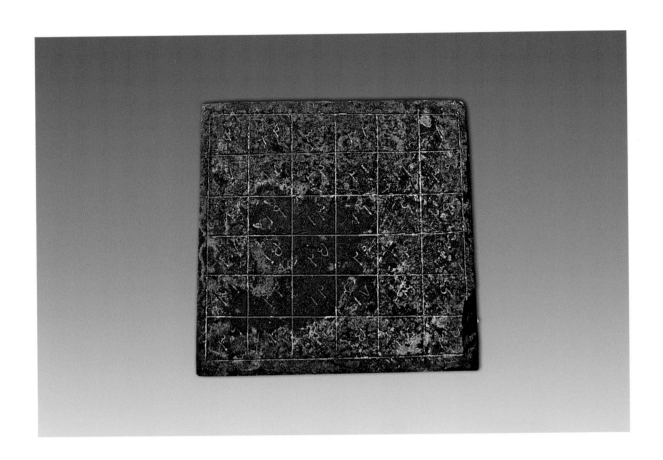

幻方

元

石质

长 15.33 厘米，宽 14.8 厘米，厚 3.21 厘米

Magic Square

Yuan Dynasty

Stone

Length 15.33 cm/ Width 14.8 cm/ Thickness 3.21 cm

六阶幻方，纵、横是古阿拉伯数字。幻方是一种将数字安排在正方形格子中，使每行、列和对角线上的数字和都相等的方法。在古代，幻方被视为神奇之物，压在房基下，作为辟邪、防灾物品。河北省张北县馒头营乡元中都中心大殿遗址出土。

元中都博物馆藏

This magic square has six grades ordered with ancient Arabic numerals. On a square, numerals are skillfully set in each block, with equal sum in each line, column and diagonal. In the old days, a square, regarded as having some mystical power, were laid under a house foundation to expel evil spirits and misfortunes. This one was excavated from the former site of the main hall of Yuanzhongdu Site at Mantouying Town, Zhangbei County, Hebei Province.

Preserved in Yuanzhongdu Museum

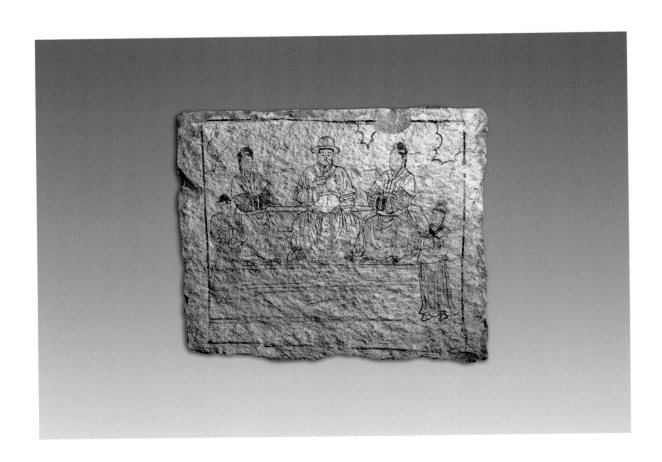

夫妇并坐图石版画

元

石质

宽 90 厘米，高 77 厘米，厚 15 厘米

Stone Engraving of a Couple Sitting Together

Yuan Dynasty

Stone

Width 90 cm/ Height 77 cm/ Thickness 15 cm

画面中央三人并坐。一男端坐居中，长圆脸，大耳，长须，头戴黄色圆顶宽檐帽，外穿右衽宽袖长袍，左手扶膝，右手端高足杯。其左、右各坐身着相同服饰，双手插袖，神态相近的女人。其左侧女人与男主距离较近。男、女侍者各一，分立两侧。

山西博物院藏

In the center of the stone engraving sit three people, with a man in the very middle who has a long round face with big ears and long beard, a yellow broad brimmed hat and a right-fastening long sleeve robe. His left hand is on his knees and his right hand is holding a stem cup. On both of his sides are sitting two women in the same clothes and almost the same posture with their hands in the sleeves. The woman on the left is closer to the man. A male attendant and a female attendant are waiting on either side of the three people.

Preserved in Shanxi Museum

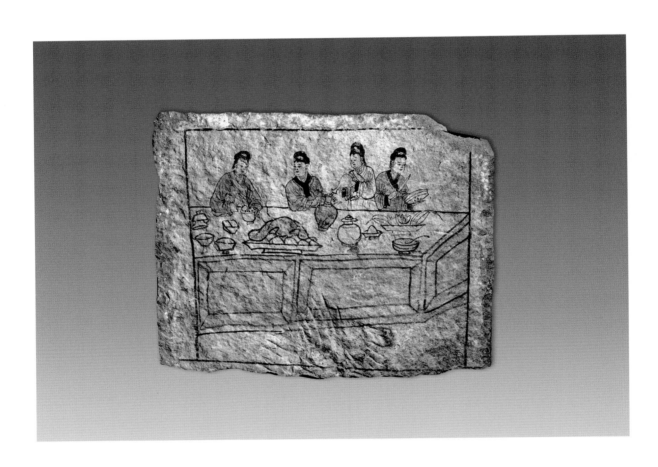

备宴图石版画

元

石质

宽 90 厘米，高 86 厘米，厚 12 厘米

Stone Engraving of Preparing for a Feast

Yuan Dynasty

Stone

Width 90 cm/ Height 86 cm/ Thickness 12 cm

画面中央有长方形案台，案台上有托盘、捣臼、高足杯、钵、盖罐等物。桌后立侍女4名，长圆脸，黑髻，分别做切食、倒酒、抚瓶、研磨等动作。

山西博物院藏

In the center of the stone engraving is a rectangular table on which trays, a mortar and pestle, stem cups, bowls and jars are placed. Behind the table stand four maids with long round faces and black hair. They are busy cutting food, pouring wine, holding the bottle or grinding.

Preserved in Shanxi Museum

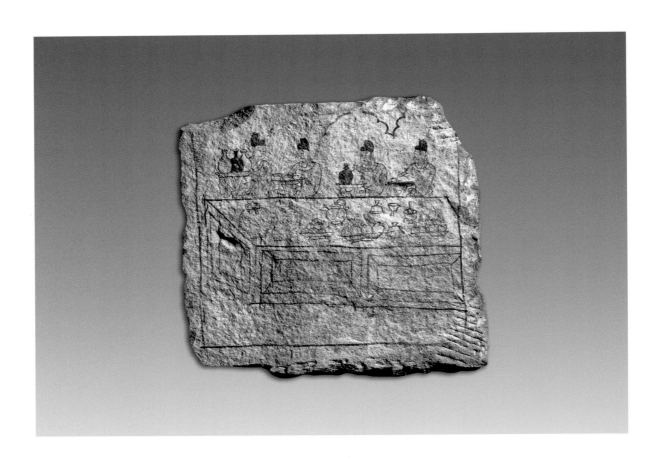

备宴图石版画

元

石质

宽 93 厘米，高 75 厘米，厚 12 厘米

Stone Engraving of Preparing for a Feast

Yuan Dynasty

Stone

Width 93 cm/ Height 75 cm/ Thickness 12 cm

画面中央有长方形案台，案台上有托盘、捣
臼、高足杯、执壶、盖罐等物。桌后立男侍4名，
长圆脸，头戴黑帽。双手捧托盘，盘中分别
置玉壶春瓶3个、碗3个、嘟噜瓶2个、肉
食1份，做进献状。

山西博物院藏

In the center of the stone engraving is a
rectangular table on which trays, a mortar and
pestle, stem cups, kettles and jars are placed.
Behind the table stand four male attendants
with long round faces and black hats. They are
in the gesture of offering food by holding trays
on which three Yuhuchun-style bottles, three
bowls, two dulu-style bottles and a meat dish
are placed.

Preserved in Shanxi Museum

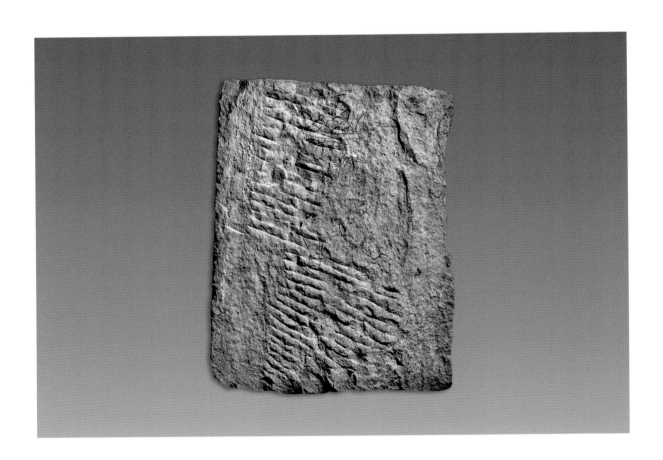

献宴图石版画

元

石质

宽 67 厘米，高 83 厘米，厚 8 厘米

Stone Engraving of Offering Food at a Feast

Yuan Dynasty

Stone

Width 67 cm/ Height 83cm/ Thickness 8 cm

画面中一身着黄色短衫，袖口紧束男子，头顶一个大托盘，盘中盛满各种水果，左手托扶盘边，右手攥拳，快步急行。

山西博物院藏

A male attendant in a cuff-fastened yellow blouse is scurrying with a large tray filled with fruits on his head, with his left hand supporting the tray edge and his right hand fisting.

Preserved in Shanxi Museum

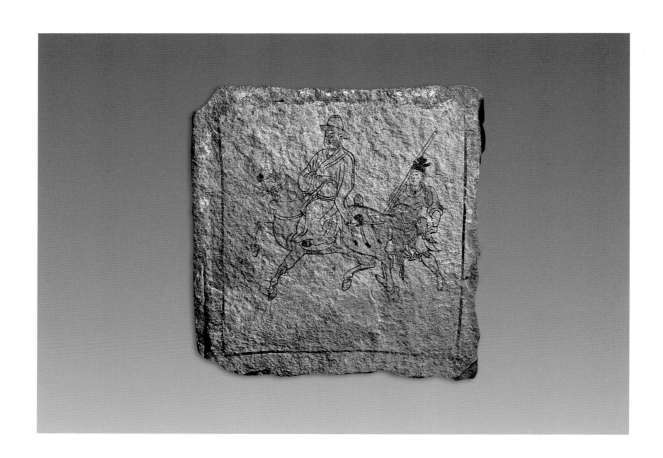

出行图石版画

元

石质

宽 73 厘米，高 76 厘米，厚 12 厘米

Stone Engraving of Traveling

Yuan Dynasty

Stone

Width 67 cm/ Height 83 cm/ Thickness 8 cm

画面中一男骑马，长圆脸，大耳，八字胡，头戴黄色圆顶宽檐帽，外穿右衽宽袖长袍，左手下垂，右手执缰，驭马疾行。马后一肩扛杖男仆，紧随其后。

山西博物院藏

A man with a long round face, big ears and a handlebar moustache is riding a horse. He wears a yellow broad brimmed hat and a right-fastening long sleeve robe. His right hand is holding the rein while his left hand is hanging. He is closely followed by a male attendant carrying a rod on his shoulder.

Preserved in Shanxi Museum

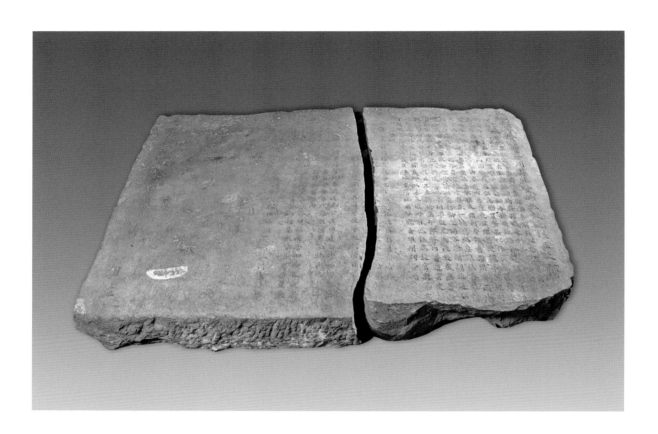

罗城县署丧葬制度碑

清

石质

宽 125 厘米，高 118 厘米，厚 13 厘米

Tablet of Official Funeral Regulations Issued by Luocheng County Government

Qing Dynasty

Stone

Width 125 cm/ Height 118 cm/ Thickness 13 cm

清代县衙仡佬族丧葬廉政制度碑刻。这块碑刻用廉政的方式告诫县官各前任和本任以及亲属等在罗城病故者，均于县城东门外从简安墓。规定用县官捐出的钱币来购买土地，加之没收土匪土地，共 100 亩，给佃户租用收取钱币，专用于县官的安葬经费。到清光绪三十四年余下银子 64 两 5 钱 2 分，谷子 800 斤，为节约经费，立碑限额购买祭品用于葬礼，为官者无论职位多高都不准超额，违者将受到府条的严惩。同时，凡清明扫墓等不准借用此经费，如确因困难必须要借的，要经集体讨论决定，由借钱人立下字据，限期归还，并加收利息每两 2 分钱，如数另刻石公布。罗城东门镇旧县署出土〔罗城民政局福利院〕。

罗城仡佬族博物馆藏

The tablet records the clean politics regulations on officials' funerals in Mulao Minority Luocheng in Qing Dynasty. This anti-corruption tablet claims that all county magistrates—the present or the former—and their relatives should be plainly buried outside the city's east gate. It says the rents of the 100-mu fields, part of which was bought with magistrates' donation and others confiscated from the outlaws, should be exclusively allocated for the funeral. In the 34th year under the reign of Emperor Guangxu in the Qing Dynasty, as is specified by the tablet, the surplus—an equivalent of 64.52 tael of silver and 800 jin of grain— is restricted only to funeral sacrificial offerings, and officials of all ranks should not overspend or they would be severely punished. The tablet also states that the special fund should not be diverted even on the Tomb-sweeping Day, and would only be loaned conditionally with a consensus agreement and a receipt by the borrower promising that he would pay back timely at an interest rate of 2%. The interest from the loan would be explicitly listed on another tablet. The tablet was excavated at the former magistrates' office, Dongmen Town, Luocheng Mulao Autonomous County, Guangxi Zhuang Autonomous Region (currently the Welfare House of the Civil Service Bureau).
Preserved in Luocheng Mulao Museum

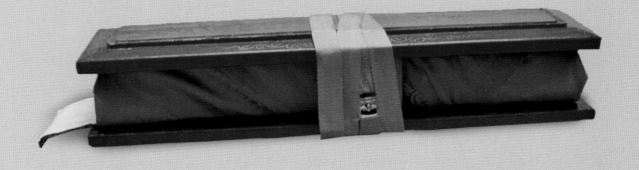

经书

现代

长 62 厘米

藏医保存医学理论的重要途径。由西藏藏医院捐赠。

成都中医药大学中医药传统文化博物馆藏

Sutra

Modern Times

Length 62 cm

Sutra is significant to preserve Tibetan medical theories. This was donated by Tibet Tibetan Hospital.

Preserved in Museum of Traditional Chinese Medicine Culture, Chengdu University of Traditional Chinese Medicine

内供颅器

清

颅骨质、金质、宝石质

长 19 厘米，宽 14 厘米，高 25.5 厘米

此件器由盖、体、托三部分组成。盖刻卷草纹、
八吉祥、莲纹，镶嵌蓝宝石花饰，口沿各嵌
一圈蓝宝石与珍珠。器体由头颅骨造成。 座
托刻卷草纹及神首像。

西藏博物馆藏

Cranium Container

Qing Dynasty

Cranium, Gold, Gem

Length 19 cm/ Width 14 cm/ Height 25.5 cm

The container consists of three parts—the lid,
the body and the saucer. The lid has rolling
grass-shaped grains, lotus-shaped grains, with
sapphires-inlaid flower decorations on it and
sapphires and pearls inlaid along its mouth.
The body is made of cranium and the saucer
is carved in rolling grass-shaped grains and
Buddha heads-shaped grains.

Preserved in Tibet Museum

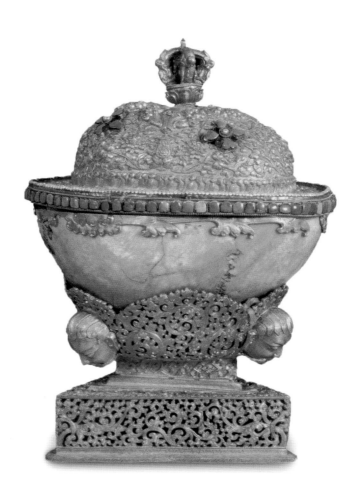

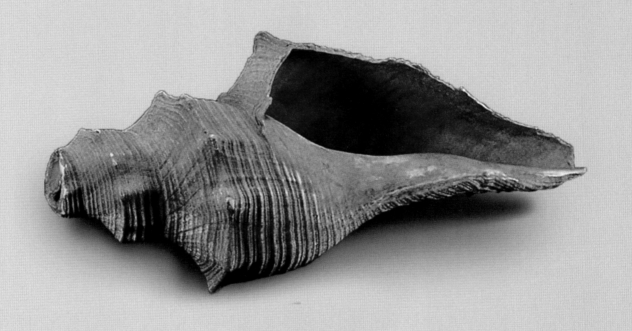

螺号

清

长 30 厘米

用海螺壳做的号角，其声响亮悦耳。蒙医进入关内行医用的行头。在陕西澄城征集。

陕西医史博物馆藏

Shell Trumpet

Qing Dynasty

Length 30 cm

The shell-made trumpet blows a nice tune. Mongolian doctors used this when they went inside Shanhaiguan Pass area to do medical practices. It was collected in Chengcheng County, Shaanxi Province.

Preserved in Shaanxi Museum of Medical History

蒙医药包

清

内有一些羊皮革质的装药小袋，每一小袋上
各书所装之药末名。蒙医草原巡诊所用。

中国医史博物馆藏

Mongolian Medical Bag

Qing Dynasty

Inside the bag there are some small sheepskin
bags which were used for containing medicines.
On each small bag, the name of medicine is
written. It was used by Mongolian doctors when
they made their rounds of visits.

Preserved in Chinese Medical History Museum

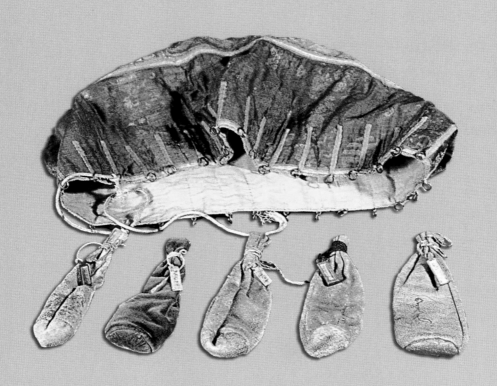

牛角

清

长 10 厘米

藏族用于拔火罐的器具。由民间征集。

　　成都中医药大学中医药传统文化博物馆藏

Ox Horn

Qing Dynasty

Length 10 cm

This ox horn was used for cupping by the Tibetans. It was collected from a private owner. Preserved in Museum of Traditional Chinese Medicine Culture, Chengdu University of Traditional Chinese Medicine

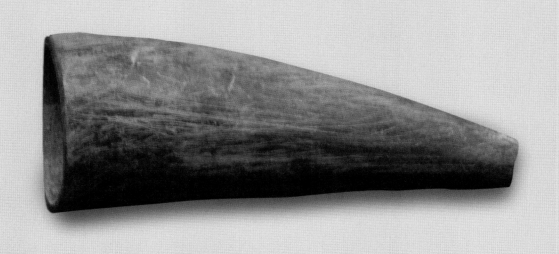

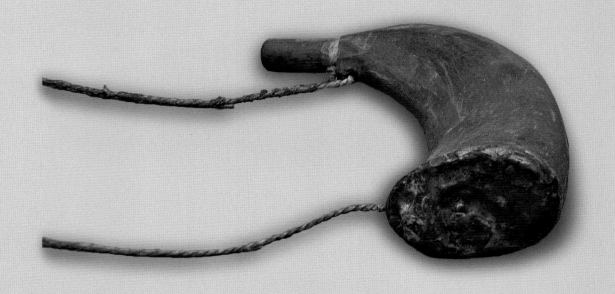

药瓶

民国时期

牛角质

长 22 厘米

牛角制，角端以木塞做盖。底与颈各钻一孔，有麻绳各一条，穿在孔中。盛药器具。由民间征集。

成都中医药大学中医药传统文化博物馆藏

Medicine Bottle

Republican Period

Ox Horn

Length 22 cm

The medicine bottle is made of ox horn and is used to keep the medicine instruments. It has a wood bung in the thinner end and two thrilled holes both in the bottom and in the bottleneck. There is a hemp rope through each hole. This bottle was collected from a private owner.

Preserved in Museum of Traditional Chinese Medicine Culture, Chengdu University of Traditional Chinese Medicine

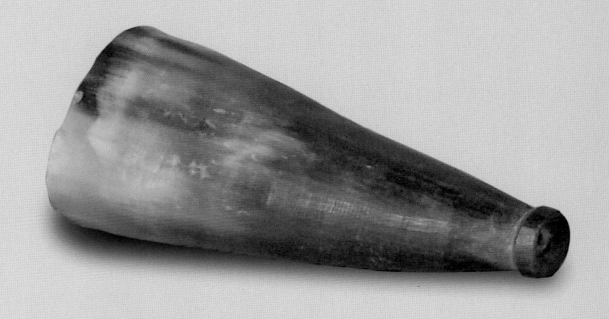

牛角吸筒

近现代

角质

长 9.8 厘米，大口径 5 厘米，小口径 1.4 厘米，
壁厚 0.5~1.1 厘米

角状，为牛角制成空心漏斗状，用处广泛。
医用。保存基本完好。

中华医学会 / 上海中医药大学医史博物馆藏

Ox Horn Suction Tube

Modern Times

Ox Horn

Length 9.8 cm/ Maximum Mouth Diameter
5 cm/ Minimum Mouth Diameter 1.4 cm/
Thickness 0.5~1.1 cm

Made of ox horn and in the shape of a funnel,
this hollow tube was used for a variety of
purposes, including medical purpose. It is still
well preserved.

Preserved in Chinese Medical Association/
Museum of Chinese Medicine, Shanghai
University of Traditional Chinese Medicine

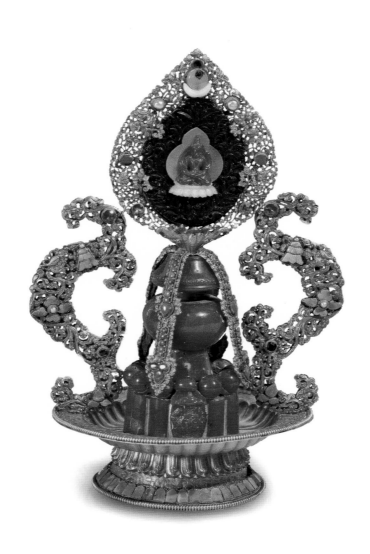

珊瑚长寿瓶

19 世纪

珊瑚质、金质、宝石质

宽 17 厘米，高 25 厘米

托盘镶嵌宝石一周，瓶身以红珊瑚为主体雕成宝塔形，桃形钮盖中央嵌有无量寿佛。整器均装饰有莲瓣纹和卷草纹饰。长寿瓶是藏传佛教举行灌顶仪式时必备的法器之一，也是无量寿佛的标志。

西藏博物馆藏

Coral-shaped Bottle of Longevity

19th Century

Coral, Gold, Gem

Width 17 cm/ Height 25 cm

The rim of the saucer is inlaid with gems, the pagoda-shaped body part is made of red coral, and the Buddha of Infinite Life is inlaid in the middle of the peach-shaped lid. There are lotus-petal-shaped grains and rolling grass-shaped grains all over the bottle. Bottle of Longevity is one of the requisite ritual items used in the Tibetan Buddhist Abhisheka. It is also a symbol of the Buddha of Infinite Life.

Preserved in Tibet Museum

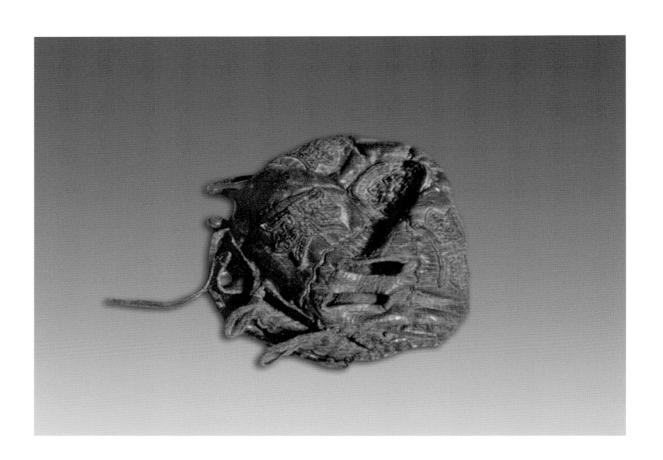

皮质碗套

20 世纪

皮质

宽 13.6 厘米，高 21 厘米

Leather Bowl Wrap

20th Century

Leather

Width 13.6 cm/ Height 21 cm

明代以后，瓷器作为一种贵重物品大量传入西藏，成为西藏上层人物身份、权力的象征。为便于携带，避免在长途跋涉中发生破损，西藏有特制的皮质碗套。套身有可以穿绳子的方孔耳环，以便于穿绳携带。

西藏博物馆藏

After the founding of the Ming Dynasty, porcelain was introduced into Tibet as a precious article and soon became a symbol of the nobility's status and power. In order to keep porcelain from being broken when carrying them in the long journey, Tibetans made the leather bowl wrap. There are square hole earrings for ropes on the wrap, which makes it easier to be carried.

Preserved in Tibet Museum

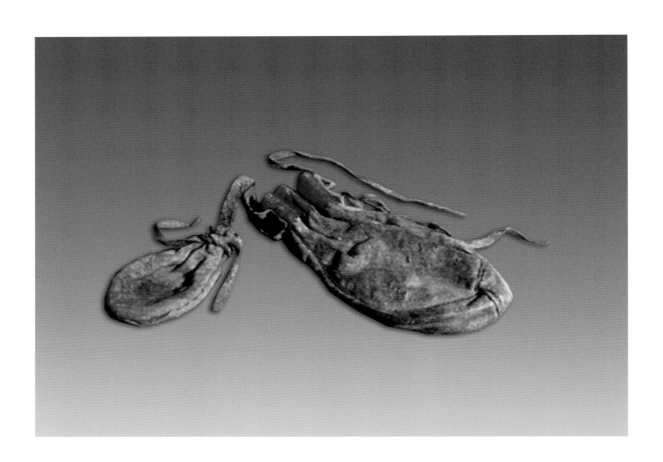

皮质茶盐袋

20 世纪

皮质

直径 20 厘米

Leather Tea and Salt Bag

20th Century

Leather

Diameter 20 cm

盛装茶盐袋子，造型美观耐用，是藏族人民日常生活中不可或缺的重要组成部分，是研究西藏文化、生活、习俗变迁发展的重要历史见证。

西藏博物馆藏

As an absolutely necessary daily life article for Tibetans, this well-designed bag was used to keep tea and salt. It also helps the historians a great deal in their researches into the development of Tibetan culture, life and custom.

Preserved in Tibet Museum

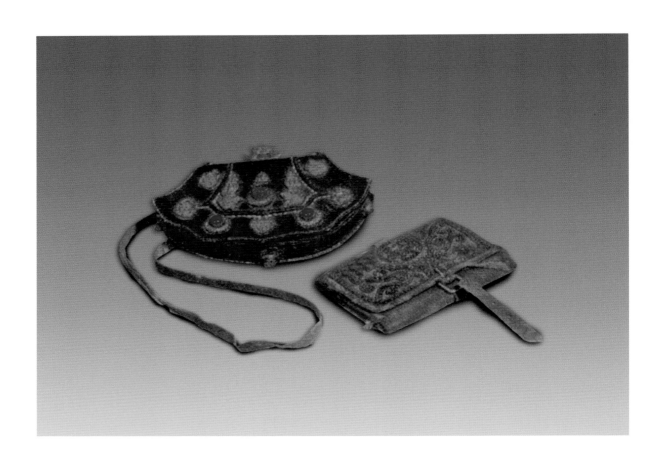

牛皮针线包

20 世纪初

牛皮质

最长 22.5 厘米

Cowhide Workboxes

Early 20th Century

Cowhide Leather

Maximum Length 22.5 cm

左为花瓣形，长带便于携带。右为长方形，无带。藏族生活用具。实用性强，造型别致，充分展示了藏族人民独特的民俗风情。

西藏博物馆藏

The flower-shaped one on the left has a long strap which is handy for carrying. The oblong one has no strap. They were used by Tibetans as daily life articles. They both have chic design and strong practicality, which fully display the unique culture and custom of Tibetans.

Preserved in Tibet Museum

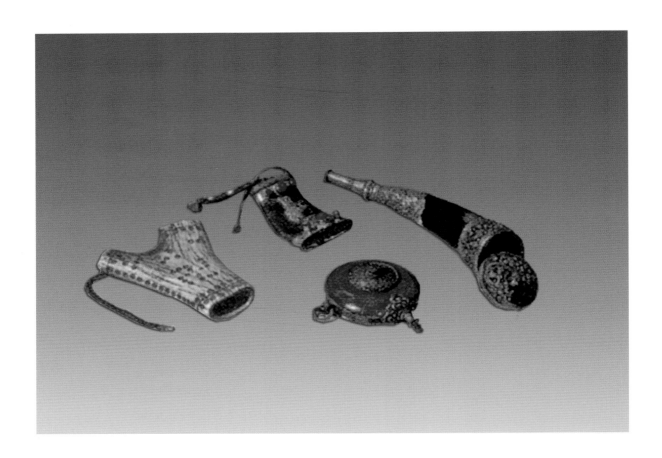

鼻烟壶

19 世纪

鹿角质、牛角质、木质、银质、玉质

最长 28.4 厘米

Snuff Bottle

19th Century

Antler, Ox Horn, Wood, Silver, Jade

Maximum Length 28.4 cm

藏式鼻烟壶，有角质、木质、银质、玉质等。

雕琢精美，依形而雕，质朴润滑，造型别致。

西藏博物馆藏

The Tibetan style snuff bottle is made of antler, ox horn, wood, silver, jade and others. Elaborately sculptured according to the shape of the raw material, it is unadorned in the quality, lubricant in hand feeling and chic in design.

Preserved in Tibet Museum

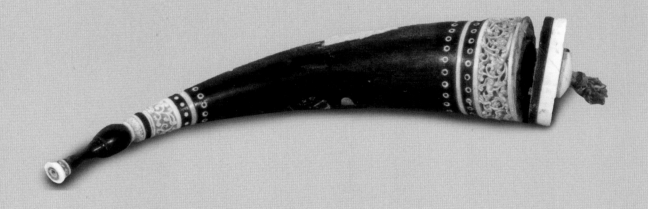

镶象牙角质鼻烟壶

19 世纪

角质、象牙质

口径 4.5 厘米，长 21 厘米

角状形，镶象牙，雕琢精美，角尖钻孔用作壶嘴。

西藏博物馆藏

Ivory-inlaid Horny Snuff Bottle

19th Century

Ox Horn, Ivory

Mouth Diameter 4.5 cm/ Length 21 cm

The elaborately sculptured snuff bottle is in the shape of a horn and is ivory-inlaid. The drill hole at the tip was utilized as the spout.

Preserved in Tibet Museum

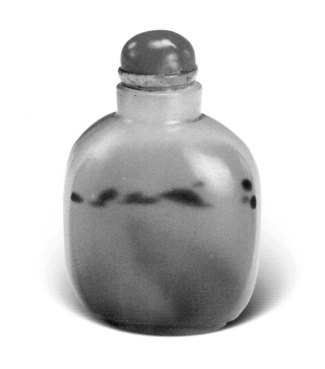

玛瑙鼻烟壶

清

玛瑙

高 7.7 厘米

用于装药。

内蒙古博物院藏

Agate Snuff Bottle

Qing Dynasty

Jade

Height 7.7 cm

It was used to store medicine.

Preserved in Inner Mongolia Museum

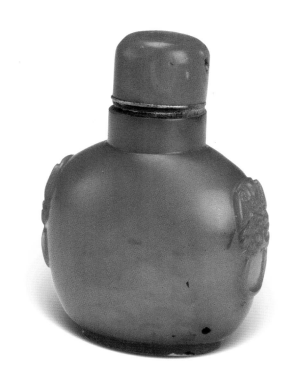

玛瑙鼻烟壶

清

玛瑙

高 8.7 厘米

用于装药。

内蒙古博物院藏

Agate Snuff Bottle

Qing Dynasty

Jade

Height 8.7 cm

It was used to store medicine.

Preserved in Inner Mongolia Museum

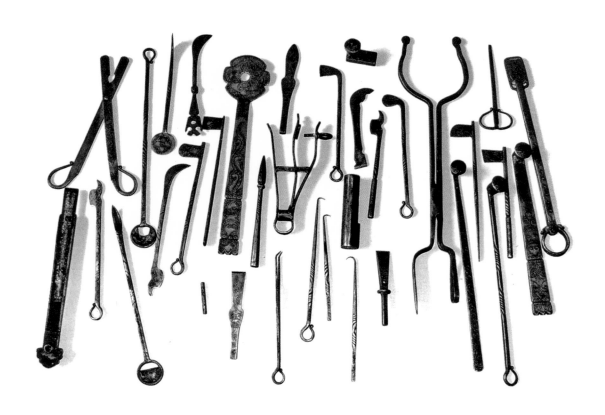

藏医手术器械

35 件，含镊子、刀、剪子、止血钳等手术器械。

张建青藏

Tibetan Surgical Instruments

This set consists of 35 pieces of surgical instruments, including knives, scissors, tweezers and forceps.

Collected by Zhang Jianqing

索 引

（馆藏地按拼音字母排序）

Index

参考文献

[1] 李经纬 . 中国古代医史图录 [M]. 北京：人民卫生出版社，1992.

[2] 傅维康，李经纬，林昭庚 . 中国医学通史：文物图谱卷 [M]. 北京：人民卫生出版社，2000.

[3] 和中浚，吴鸿洲 . 中华医学文物图集 [M]. 成都：四川人民出版社，2001.

[4] 上海中医药博物馆 . 上海中医药博物馆馆藏珍品 [M]. 上海：上海科学技术出版社，2013.

[5] 西藏自治区博物馆 . 西藏博物馆 [M]. 北京：五洲传播出版社，2005.

[6] 崔乐泉 . 中国古代体育文物图录：中英文本 [M]. 北京：中华书局，2000.

[7] 张金明，陆雪春 . 中国古铜镜鉴赏图录 [M]. 北京：中国民族摄影艺术出版社，2002.

[8] 文物精华编辑委员会 . 文物精华 [M]. 北京：文物出版社，1964.

[9] 谭维四 . 湖北出土文物精华 [M]. 武汉：湖北教育出版社，2001.

[10] 常州市博物馆 . 常州文物精华 [M]. 北京：文物出版社，1998.

[11] 镇江博物馆 . 镇江文物精华 [M]. 合肥：黄山书社，1997.

[12] 贵州省文化厅，贵州省博物馆 . 贵州文物精华 [M]. 贵阳：贵州人民出版社，2005.

[13] 徐良玉 . 扬州馆藏文物精华 [M]. 南京：江苏古籍出版社，2001.

[14] 昭陵博物馆，陕西历史博物馆 . 昭陵文物精华 [M]. 西安：陕西人民美术出版社，1991.

[15] 南通博物苑 . 南通博物苑文物精华 [M]. 北京：文物出版社，2005.

[16] 邯郸市文物研究所 . 邯郸文物精华 [M]. 北京：文物出版社，2005.

[17] 张秀生，刘友恒，聂连顺，等 . 中国河北正定文物精华 [M]. 北京：文化艺术出版社，1998.

[18] 陕西省咸阳市文物局 . 咸阳文物精华 [M]. 北京：文物出版社，2002.

[19] 安阳市文物管理局 . 安阳文物精华 [M]. 北京：文物出版社，2004.

[20] 深圳市博物馆 . 深圳市博物馆文物精华 [M]. 北京：文物出版社，1998.

[21]《中国文物精华》编辑委员会 . 中国文物精华（1993）[M]. 北京：文物出版社，1993.

[22] 夏路，刘永生 . 山西省博物馆馆藏文物精华 [M]. 太原：山西人民出版社，1999.

[23] 文物精华编辑委员会 . 文物精华 [M]. 文物出版社，1957.

[24] 山西博物院，湖北省博物馆 . 荆楚长歌：九连墩楚墓出土文物精华 [M]. 太原：山西人民出版社，2011.

[25] 刘广堂，石金鸣，宋建忠 . 晋国雄风：山西出土两周文物精华 [M]. 沈阳：万卷出版公司，2009.

[26] 沈君山，王国平，单迎红 . 滦平博物馆馆藏文物精华 [M]. 北京：中国文联出版社，2012.

[27] 张家口市博物馆 . 张家口市博物馆馆藏文物精华 [M]. 北京：科学出版社，2011.

[28] 浙江省文物考古研究所 . 浙江考古精华 [M]. 北京：文物出版社，1999.

[29] 故宫博物院 . 故宫雕刻珍萃 [M]. 北京：紫禁城出版社，2004.

[30] 故宫博物院紫禁城出版社 . 故宫博物院藏宝录 [M]. 上海：上海文艺出版社，1986.

[31] 首都博物馆 . 大元三都 [M]. 北京：科学出版社，2016.

[32] 新疆维吾尔自治区博物馆 . 新疆出土文物 [M]. 北京：文物出版社，1975.

[33] 王兴伊，段逸山 . 新疆出土涉医文书辑校 [M]. 上海：上海科学技术出版社，2016.

[34] 刘学春 . 刍议医药卫生文物的概念与分类标准 [J]. 中华中医药杂志，2016，31（11）:4406-4409.

[35] 上海古籍出版社 . 中国艺海 [M]. 上海：上海古籍出版社，1994.

[36] 紫都，岳鑫 . 一生必知的 200 件国宝 [M]. 呼和浩特：远方出版社，2005.

[37] 谭维四 . 湖北出土文物精华 [M]. 武汉：湖北教育出版社，2001.

[38] 张建青 . 青海彩陶收藏与鉴赏 [M]. 北京：中国文史出版社，2007.

[39] 银景琦 . 仡佬族文物 [M]. 南宁：广西人民出版社，2014.

[40] 廖果，梁峻，李经纬 . 东西方医学的反思与前瞻 [M]. 北京：中医古籍出版社，2002.

[41] 梁峻，张志斌，廖果，等 . 中华医药文明史集论 [M]. 北京：中医古籍出版社，2003.

[42] 郑蓉，庄乾竹，刘聪，等 . 中国医药文化遗产考论 [M]. 北京：中医古籍出版社，2005.